For Chris, with smiles....

You asked me which essential oils you need to have. Personally, I think this is one that should be top of your list...

> "You do not *see* anything when you experience pure consciousness; you *become* everything."
> – Sebastian Pole

All Rights Reserved. No part of this publication may be reproduced in any form or by any means, including scanning, photocopying, or otherwise without prior written permission of the copyright holder.
Copyright © 2015 Elizabeth Ashley – The Secret Healer

I sometimes think that I have no favourite oils because they are all my favourites! Every oil I spend time with amazes me, thrills me and humbles me. Without fail their healing abilities astound me, and as I open the lid of a new oil I always prepare to be both intrigued and astounded.

Nothing could have prepared me for how I would come to feel about Holy Basil. I feel like She rescued me from the precipice of madness and rocked me through one of the most terrifying nights of my life…then stole away taking the terror with her.

Look her up and without fail you will see Tulasi, as the Hindu faith calls her, described as adaptogen but there is no way you can fully comprehend the true depth of her healing. Yes, she will bring back the body into homeostasis after stress, but there is so much more. She holds the soul fast in the most shattering of moments; she is most assuredly *"The Destroyer of Demons."*

This extraordinary plant is believed by the Hindus to be the earthly embodiment of the goddess Lakshmi. It is quintessentially linked to their religious ceremonies and prayers to Vishnu, and carries the well deserved mantle *"The Queen of Medicine Herbs"*

Together, let's discover the plant which is

- Fighting many, many different cancers

- Lessening the effects of diabetes and may even be able to restore sight after diabetic retinopathy has taken hold
- Protecting mouth and teeth from infections and decay

Amongst hundreds of other complaints.

Described by Ayurvedic doctors as **sattvic**, *Ocimum sanctum* is purity itself.

Come with me and discover the oil they call *The Elixir of Life*.

Table of Contents

Table of Contents 5
Chapter 1 Holy Basil 7
   Etymology 7
   Botany 8
   Family 9
Chapter 2 The Sacred Embodiment of Lakshmi 11
   The Goddess Who Became a Plant 11
   References from Charaka Samhita 15
   Other ceremonial usages of Tulsi 18
   Prasadam 20
   Tulsi vivah, the marriage of Tulsi 21
   Rasayana 21
Chapter 3 Traditional Ayurvedic Medicine 24
   Effects on the Doshas 29
   Holy Basil Tincture 32
Chapter 4 Twenty First Century Usage of Tulasi 36
   Clinical Evidence of the Physical Effects of Holy Basil 38
   Spiritual Aspects of Holy Basil 78
   Emotional aspects of Basil 82
   Chakras 84
   Ruling Planet 86
Chapter 5 The Essential Oil 90
   Extraction 90
   Yield 90
   Safety Data 90

Distribution 91
Blending 92
How to meditate with Tulsi 92
Vibration 94
Colour 94
Musical Note 94
Recipes 96
Prayer of Gratitude 101
Authors comment 102
Resources 104
Other books in The Secret Healer Series 105
About the Author 118

Chapter 1 Holy Basil

Etymology

Tulsi is, quite simply, the most sacred plant in India. Her name means ***The Incomparable One: The one who will not tolerate or permit similarity.***

Most commonly this plant is known as *Holy Basil* in English, *Thiruthuzhai* in Tamil and *Tulasi* or *Tulsi* in Sanskrit. In some texts you might see it listed as *Vishnu Priya*, or perhaps its most visual descriptor is "Destroyer of Demons".

Correct English pronunciation is articulated as *Tool-See*.

I can't decide which version I like best so throughout the book I will flit butterfly-like between the names. By the end, hopefully we will all be multi-lingual in the tongue of Holy Basil!

The most important thing, I think to consider about Holy Basil is: it is seen, by the Hindus as **the ultimate symbol of purity**. Because it is so deeply revered by them, as the embodiment of the Goddess Lakshmi, there are a great many variations of names and customs. The plant is seen as the link between the spiritual and domestic worlds.

The Tulasi plant, as it is known in India is available and grown in two forms. These are *Dark Krishna* or *Shyama Tulsi* which has purple leaves and also white (or more accurately described as light green) basil which is known as *Rama Tulasi* or *White Tulsi*. Both Tulsi plants have a great number of properties, but it is **Shyama Tulsi that has the most medicinal prowess is most commonly the sub species worshipped by most Hindus**. You might also find *Rama Tulasi* (also called *Vana Tulasi*) which is *Ocimum gratissimum* listed by some authorities under the umbrella of Sacred Basil. In Hindi you might also see this chemotype referred to as *Hindi janglitulsi* or "forest tulsi".

More recently, in the West, Tulsi has taken on a new monicker "Sulabha" which means "The Easily Obtainable One" showing just how far its propagation and usage has now spread throughout the Western world.

Botany

Ocimum sanctum is native to India. It grows wild throughout Asia and Malaysia and can be seen growing in gardens in pots. The leaves which are ovate and slightly toothed are richly laden with essential oils. Hindu tradition is to have either nine of eleven plants growing around the front of the home or the temple to keep negativity away from the door. Throughout Asia She is recognised as the Queen of Herbs The Mother Medicine of Nature and the Elixir of Life. Holy Basil is an extraordinarily fragrant plant as the warm sun relaxes the essential oil sacs in the leaves, she releases her fragrance into the air purifying it, dissipating tension and reducing stress.

Family

Basil belongs to the Lamiaceae family, which you might see listed as Labiteae in older text books. It is the same herbaceous family that lavender, rosemary and sage belong to. It is classified here because of the way its leaves grow in opposition to each other and emerge in whorls. They have flowering tips and all parts of the plants are aromatic.

The interesting thing about the basil family is they are all female. Whilst this book focuses on Holy Basil, it is important to make the distinction here, I think between Holy Basil and the more usual basil essential oil you might see on sale which is Sweet Basil, or *Ocimum basilicum.* Although the energy of Sweet Basil is resoundingly masculine – (almost *Sergeant Major-ish* in its no messing nature) botanically speaking there is no such thing as a male basil. Over time they have evolved to self seed and pollinate and so, although there might be a few male flowers on the plant to aid the process of pollination, for the most part the Basil plant is all Woman! Most assuredly Holy Basil is more than woman...She is Goddess.

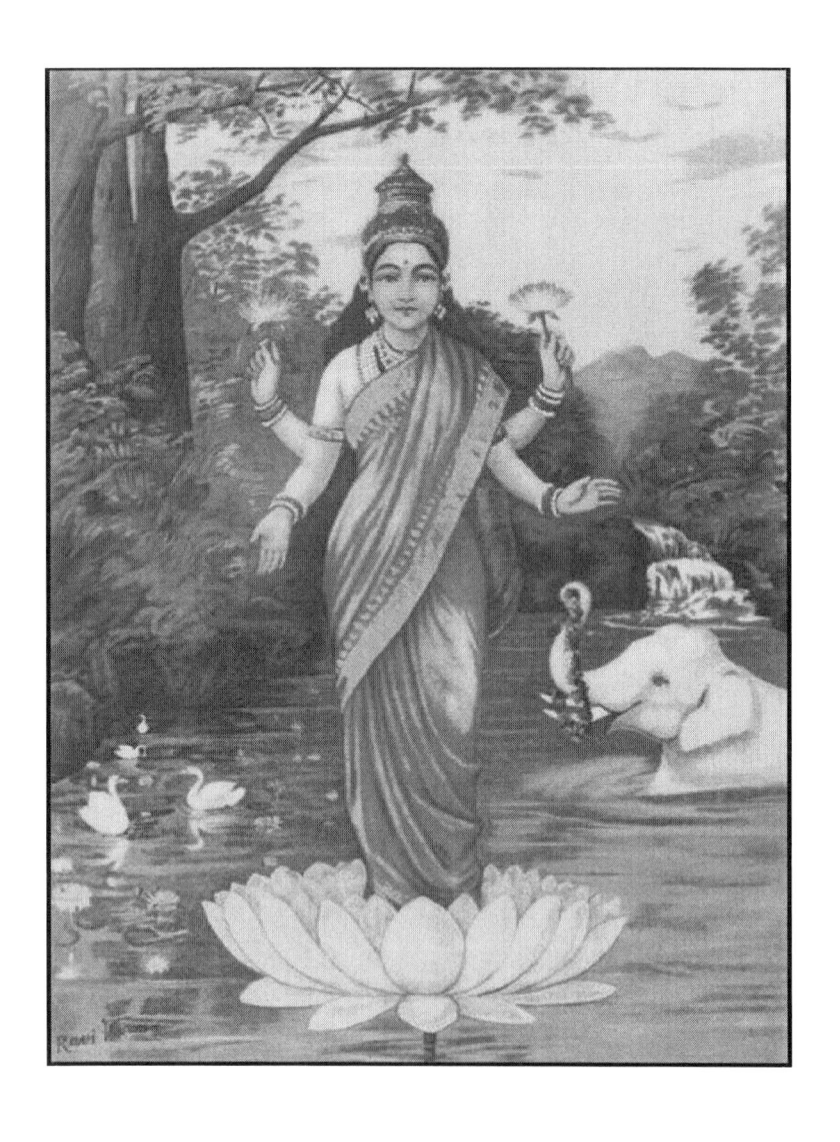

Chapter 2 The Sacred Embodiment of Lakshmi

The Goddess Who Became a Plant

Tulsi, or Tulasi is the embodiment of the Goddess Lakshmi, the Hindu goddess of wealth, love and fortune, of prosperity (both spiritual and material) and of beauty. She is the wife and the active energy of Vishnu, the Lord Preserver and Protector.

Pictorially you see Lakshmi extending four hands. In these are cradled each of the **Purusartha**, the Hindu ways of life. These are:

- **Dharma**: The duties and laws, the rightful ways of life. The term means "To hold, maintain" and has a similar connotation to the Buddhist ideal of cosmic order.
- **Kama:** This means desire, wish, longing and this embodies an enjoyment of the aesthetic in life. This might be with or without the sexual connotation.
- **Artha:** This is material, prosperity, income, security. The means of living.
- **Moksha:** Liberation, self actualisation, release.

Together the four Purusartha are seen as the route to a successful Hindu life. It follows then that because Sacred Basil is the embodiment of Lakshmi, then the plant also holds the medicine of these spiritual virtues.

According to ancient scriptures all women are the embodiment of Lakshmi. *Diwali and Sharad Purnima* are both celebrated in her name and indeed there have been archaeological discoveries showing reverence to her, as goddess, as early as the 1st millennium BCE. To this day, it is believed that no prayer to Vishnu is complete unless it is accompanied with Tulasi. For this reason then, plants are grown in Hindu houses for leaves to be offered in prayer.

Tulasi is mentioned once in the sacred collection of Hindu scriptures, the Rig Veda, beautiful ancient hymns of praise dating from around 1500-2000BCE. It is thought these are possibly the oldest religious writings in existence. Here though, according to John Muir's *Original Text on the Origin and History of the People of India. Their Religions and Institutions,* her name seems to have a different translation to contemporary references. Rather than "Goddess of Wealth" it is thought the correct attribution in the Rig Veda might be "Kindred mark or sign of auspicious fortune".

There seem to be countless myths as to how the goddess came to be housed within the plant of Holy Basil. I'll recount a couple of my favourites for you.

The earliest I can find comes from the Fourth Veda, the sacred text known as the *Arthravaveda*, dating from around 1500 BCE. Here, the birth of Lakshmi is described many times through the record. It details how a hundred Lakshmis came to Earth in the form of a mortal. Some incarnations were good and some bad. The bad were encouraged to leave. The good versions were seen to be fortune, health etc etc.

Another account has Lakshmi emerging at the point of creation of the universe and floating above the water on a lotus flower.

The most well loved version seems to be how a mortal girl Vrinder (sometimes seen as Brinder) married a demon Jalandhara. She loved her husband so much that every time he went off to battle she prayed to Lord Vishnu for his safe return. Jalandhara's powers became ever stronger, but so did his ambition and ego. Soon taking over the Earth was not enough for Jalandhara and he began to aspire for dominion over the Heavens too. Having disregard for the Shiva, Vishnu and Brahman, he insulted each of them in turn. It became clear that the only way to defeat Jalanhandra was to halt Vrinders prayers to Vishnu.

Next day when Jalandhara went off to battle with Lord Shiva, Vrinder prayed, but began to sense someone was in the room with her. When she opened her eyes, the form of her husband stood before her announcing "I have done it. I have defeated Lord Shiva", unbeknownst to her, Lord Vishnu was instead speaking to her in Jalanhandra's form.

Vrinder stopped her prayers and went to prepare celebrations for her husband. As the prayers ceased, Jalanhandra's power subsided. Lord Shiva plunged a sword into his heart.

Vrinder sensed the change in her world and seemed to feel her husband slip away. She demanded of the man before her "Who are you? What have you done with my husband?" Lord Vishnu ended the illusion and stood before her with sad eyes and apologised to her for what he had had to do. He explained that Jalandhara's power had come from her love of Lord Vishnu and it had been *her* that had made him so great. Sadly though, she had neglected her duty. As she began to see him becoming more maniacal and bad, Vishnu explained, she should have stopped him in his tracks.

Vrinder was heartbroken and died there, before her Lord.

When Lord Shiva and Lord Brahman came down to Earth they found Lord Vishnu bent over her in grief. "Don't mourn for her" they said "for she will be reincarnated as Tulasi, the plant with more medicinal properties than any other on Earth."

And so it was that Vrinder, the mortal, became wife and consort to Lord Vishnu and became embodied by the most Holy Basil.

In Vaishnavism, one form of Hinduism, there is a beautiful story of how the oceans of milk were churned in the fight between the asuras (demons) and the gods. When the gods won, Dhanvatri (the physician god and god of Ayurvedic medicine) raised up from the waves with amrita in hand for the gods (Amrita: some translations say immortality, others relate nectar). As Dhanvatri shed a happy tear, it fell onto amrita and Tulasi was formed. Visitors to Kerala and Tamil Nadu can still visit temples to Dhanvatri where ayurvedic medicine is practiced.

There is also mention of Tulasi in the ancient writings Charaka Samhita. This along along with the Sushruta Samhita form the basis of Ayurvedic medicine and they date from around 900 BC- 600BCE. Here it is described *as a life saving herb, an "Elixir of Life" that promotes longevity.*

The Sushrata samhita, for the most part relates to surgical instruction where the charaka samhita is far more concerned with using plants as medicine. For this reason Charaka Samhita is now referred to as the main text of Ayurveda. When put together, the samhitas are massive tomes. An English translation from 1996 ran to a rather intimidating 2700 pages!

References from Charaka Samhita

- It is listed as anti-dyspneic (shortness of breath associated with heart disease)

- *"Women say that during this month because of appearance of hairs in the fetus, they cause burning sensation in the mother but Lord Atreya says that due to pressure of the fetus V, P and K [vata, pitta, and kapha] reaching into the chest give rise to burning sensation, then itching which in turn causes kikkisa (streaking of the skin). To ameliorate this condition, she should take in food times butter processed with sweet drugs along with the decoction of kola (jujube). Besides, her breast areola should be massaged gently with the paste of sandal and lotus stalk; or the powder of dhataki, mustard and madhuka; or the paste of kutaja, arjaka seeds, musta and haridra; or the paste of nimba, kola, tulasi and manjistha; or triphala mixed with blood of prsat (spotted deer), deer and rabbit, massage with oil cooked with karavira leaves and sprinkling with water processed with jati and madhuka should be applied"*

"The following [paste] should be used for anointing on the body (which should have been prior-ly smeared with oil). By this formula itching, boils, urticarial patches, skin diseases and various types of edema are alleviated: equal parts of each- kustha, both types of haridra, tulasi, patola, nimba, aswagandha, devadaru, sigru, sarsapa, tumburu, dhanyaka, kaivarta [,] mustaka, candana Powder all the above together. + buttermilk Grind all of the above together."

Many Ayurvedic scripts also suggest adding Tulsi to bathwater to strengthen against colds as an herbal tea, dried powder, fresh leaf, or mixed with Honey or Ghee

Other ceremonial usages of Tulsi

It is written that for the finest of offerings to Vishu you should serve Tulasi with some pulp of sandalwood and place it on the lotus flowers of his feet.

Hindu Devotees wear beautiful Rosary Prayer necklaces which are made by stringing beads onto the stalks. Traditionally a necklace will have 108 beads and the bracelet 27. The wood of the Tulsi is thought to imbue devotion and each bead is used for counting the cycles of breath in prayer.

In a Hindu household, Holy Basil is often planted into its own stage in courtyards and in front of homes. Devotees are encouraged to grow and care for their plants so they always have fresh leaves to offer up in prayer. Only women though are allowed the honour of watering or caring for the plant. A Tulsi-vrindavan (see picture) is considered to be a place of pilgrimage.

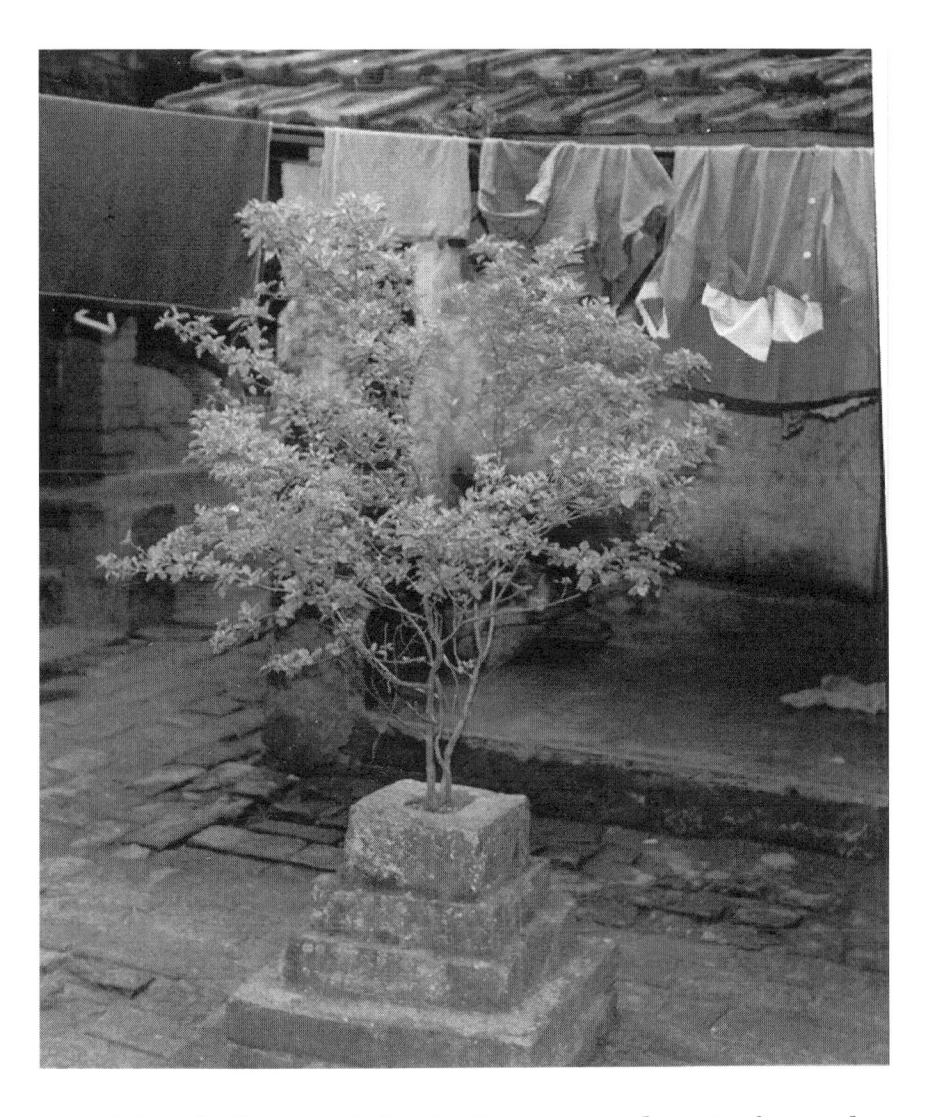

A *Tulsi-vrindavan* sitting in the courtyard, part of everyday Hindu culture.

Prasadam

Tulsi is the first offering in prasadam.

Prasada is mentioned in some of the earliest texts of Rig Veda. Originally denoting the *material* offering, it was aligned to the spiritual experience the gods and sages underwent when they were bestowed with gifts. Later the name began to take on the meaning of the actual *ritual* of offering.

Offerings are made to the deity in the form of fruits, herbs and sweets, this is known as *naivedya*.

The deity then takes a small taste of the goods and this is referred to as *boghya*. Then these blessed goods are either eaten by the devotee, or shared amongst the others in the temple. This partaking of blessed foods is Prasad. Some devotees strictly maintain only eating food that is Prasad, but standard Hindu practice is to eat blessed food only on special occasions.

There seems to be no ideal number of Tulsi leaves required in the offering, only that the same number be picked each day at the same time. Then She is believed to fall into line (and generate enough leaves to continue) with this regularity. When fresh leaves are unavailable, then according to much loved swami *Srila Prabhupada* dried leaves will serve just as well.

Tulsi vivah, the marriage of Tulsi

The sacred celebration of Tulsi vivah signifies the marriage of Tulasi to Vishnu or his avatar (the human form descended to Earth) Krishna. The actual date of celebration varies from region to region but signifies the end of the monsoon season and the beginning of the Hindu wedding season.

The ceremony itself resembles a traditional wedding and can be performed in homes and in temples. The Tulsi plant is placed in the middle of the courtyard and is decorated with sari fabrics and necklaces, beside her sits a brass representation of Vishnu. Around them is spun a cotton thread to denote their wedding vows. Prasad of nuts, sweets and sugar cane are offered. For the most part the ritual of Tulsi vivah is performed by women and there is a spectacular video of this being performed in the resources section at the back of this book.

Rasayana

The term *Rasayana* comes from the very earliest Ayurvedic texts and its English translation from the Sanskrit means "The Science of Lengthening Life". In texts later than the 8th Century the meaning takes on a slightly different slant and it becomes the name of Indian Alchemy.

This term is sometimes interchanged with the more specific name *Rasaśāstra,* रसशास्तर which pertains to "The Science of

Mercury" because many of the treatments employed at the time did in fact use mercury, but also there were a number of medicinal tinctures too. Most notably amongst the herbs used was Holy Basil but other ingredients often included gem stones, coral, pearls and precious metals.

Recorded history from a Persian chemist and physician from the 11th Century, tells of how, in India a very different type of alchemy took place from the rest of the World. Where the Arabs focused on such activities as creating dyes or even processing metals, India were firmly focused on healing with plants. Abū Rayhān Bīrūnī goes on to relate *""They have a science similar to alchemy which is quite peculiar to them. They call it Rasâyana, a word composed with rasa, i.e., gold. It means an art which is restricted to certain operations, drugs, and compound medicines, most of which are taken from plants. Its principles restore the health of those who were ill beyond hope, and give back youth to fading old age..."*

The focus of this school of thought was to achieve Moksha, liberation...through mercury. The objective of Moksha is to achieve transformation from mortal to immortal. Strangely we now find that Holy Basil contains high levels of magnesium....and mercury!

Rasayana therapy is thought to enrich rasa with nutrients to attain a lustrous complexion, youthfulness and health. It improves voice, aids longevity, memory, & intelligence. It lengthens health and preserves youthfulness. Rasayana develops physique and sensory organs to the best of their capacity. It imbues mastery over phonetics, respectability and brilliance.

No-one can fail to notice the exquisite beauty of a Hindu woman when she is dressed up in her regalia and when you absorb the ideals of rasayana you can see just how effectively their radiant secret does indeed shine through.

Holy Basil is considered to be rasayana.

Chapter 3 Traditional Ayurvedic Medicine

Ayurvedic medicine courses through the veins of India. The medicinal and spiritual properties of a plant are almost not seen as separate things there, more extensions of the same. The knowledge of the plants has been passed from generation to generation and those details which have defied inscription onto paper are still firmly ingrained in local culture.

In amongst all the scientific research, I found a lovely paper into attitudes of mothers in Delhi about how they preferred to treat their children when they have measles. Of the 387 ladies surveyed 97% said they liked to feed the ailing kids with traditional foods to encourage healing. The favourite dish was cows' milk and kitchdi (a delicious moong dahl and rice dish, which contains cumin, turmeric and asofoetida). 95.1% said they would apply medicinal leaves to the sores. Traditional herbs chosen by them are *Laung* (cloves), Tulsi leaves and Kishmish (raisins) in that order.

Considering that they are working on information passed through generations for the last 5000 years you might be astounded to see just how accurate a prescription clinical trials are showing these to be. The active constituent seemingly harnessing most of the magic in Tulsi is called Euganol which is found in even larger quantities in cloves! The sad detail uncovered by this study is that worryingly only 77.5% of the women surveyed were aware that the dangerous illness of measles is an infectious disease.

I have also been struck by the sharp divide in how different sites on the internet view the ways Tulasi should to be used. Those who revere her for prayer seem to be entirely offended by the idea that the herb might be sold for medicinal or culinary purposes, because how could someone think of exploiting her sanctity for profit?

That said, another of her names is the Mother of Medicinal Plants, and whilst many other plants might have maybe, half a dozen uses attributed to them, it is said that Tulasi has literally hundreds.

In Vetiver: An Ayurvedic Medicine we took a cursory look at the doshas, vata, pitta, kapha. Here I'd like to look even further back into the myths of Avurveda, to their stories of the dawn of the Universe.

It is said that before the beginning there was a vast expanse of nothingness. In Sanskrit this is referred to as *Shunyakasha*. It was like an empty page just waiting to be written or drawn upon, entirely full of potential. From this void of potential sprung a desire for creation, and the first sound of consciousness vibrated through the ether. Its sound was AUM.

The sound then split into tremendous, opposing forces.

- **Purusha** – A masculine energy of the origins of consciousness. This was unchanging and divine energy believed to be representative of Lord Shiva.
- **Prakriti** – A primordial divine feminine energy, believed to be the energy of the goddess Shakti

Prakriti is the force of creation that exists in all things. Whilst magnificent, this energy is nothing without the tattvas (we might more readily call them the elements). These are required to bring *anything* into being.

The five **tattvas**, *earth, air, fire, water and ether*, galvanise prakriti into being.

They require the *gunas* to anchor them in reality rather than them simply floating in cosmic nothingness.

Beautiful, isn't it….but very confusing I find, until you bring the gunas into the mix. Suddenly that which has been nebulous begins to become tangible.

There isn't really a direct English translation for guna. Consider: *string, thread, strand, virtue, merit, excellence, peculiarity, attribute, property* or for me the closest feels like *quality.*

There are three gunas

- **Sattva** – goodness, constructive, harmony, equilibrium, balance, gentleness, purity, clarity

- **Rajas** – Passion, active, confused, anger, restlessness, anxiety, untamed emotions
- **Tamas** – Darkness, destructive, chaotic, inertia, laziness, sloth and ignorance.

It is said the gunas were, are and always will be present in all things in the world. All gunas are considered to be equal but sattva is the most rarified of the three.

So we might describe them as being:

Sattvic – being purified

Rajasika – Excitable

Tamasika -Indifferent

Tulsi is considered to be sattvic.

For a plant to hold the title of **sattvic** it must meet certain criteria. It must not be contaminated and should not spread disease or evil in the world. It should purify its surroundings. When it is eaten the person eating it must feel as if they are consuming the very purest food. It must not weaken the mind or challenge the equilibrium. (*Which means if a plant has aphrodisiac properties like vetiver does, or it can be used as a drug, then it cannot be considered to be sattvic*). When it is picked from the plant the mind should be steady, calm and peaceful and here, I think it is useful to add, there is an I-Thou relationship as the aroma of the plant exudes an aura of calm when you enter its space to pick the leaves.

Whilst there are few detailed accounts into the spiritual dimensions of Tulsi it is helpful to imagine some sattvic properties which probably explain it better.

Its energy is light and warming. It is pure and always moving. It is transparent and diffuses upwards. It is joyful, light and simple.

The sattvic mind is clear and content. It is inspired and concentrated. Most of all it is accepting. It is attached to knowledge and happiness. It is always steady. It finds delight internally without having to turn the attention out into the world for excitement and stimulation. Once it lands in one place it will remain there for great lengths of time. The friendships it builds are long lasting, bright, vibrant and loyal.

Holy basil holds a mirror up to the soul and helps to make soul connections. Because the mirror is so clean and pure, it becomes easy to see parts of you reflected in other people's souls. Reasons for connections become far clearer and relationships are able to move onto a more soul enriching pathway.

Staring into the mirror it is easier to see our divine source reflected. Inspiration spills forth. Beautiful poetry, heartfelt songs, and magical music all pour from sattvic energy.

Its emotions are devotion, peace and humility. The gentle smile of cheerfulness; of contentment and love.

In the body we can expect lightness, composure and energy.

Sattvic *environments* are clean, fresh, tranquil, harmonious, cooperative and green (environmentally speaking rather than the colour!)

Food that is sattvic is fresh, light, easily digestible and calming. Most of all, it is abundant with the universal light-giving source of prana.

When someone works with sattvic energy they do it with no attachment to the end result, so we should think **without reward** and ***faith in charity***. In the *Bhagavada Gita* it is explained that all three gunas are chains, (albeit made of gold, silver and steel) but laying attachment aside raises the consciousness above all three gunas (even sattvic guna) and it points the attention towards liberation and moksha.

Effects on the Doshas

Holy Basil is **invigorating to Kapha dosha**.

The attributes of kapha are heavy, slow, steady, solid, cold, soft, sticky, slimy and oily.

If you consider that kapha is considered to be earth and water elements combined, (which, of course, is heavy mud) it helps you to picture some of the afflictions connected with this.

Kapha governs the connective tissues of the body, the ligaments, muscles, sinews, fat and bone.

As explained in Vetiver and Ayurvedic Medicine; the doshas are attributes that pertain to the physical and mental characteristics if a person as will as actual symptoms. So a kapha type is a very calm and steady person. Solid and stable we might say. They sleep well and have good digestion. They have lovely clear skin and bright eyes. Being married to the text book kapha I feel qualified to say strong, silent types, they tend not to say very much either.

When kapha energy goes out of balance though, they get slower. Digestion becomes sluggish. They begin to sleep too much. They gain weight and might start to suffer from water retention. Allergies can become a problem as can diabetes, asthma and often depression. Emotionally too, you will see stubbornness and a desire to ignore the things going on around them.

So…

Physical attributes of Holy Basil on kapha dosha

Problems pertaining to connective tissue

- Sprains, strains and pulled ligaments
- Retention of fluids from injury such as inflammation, bursitis, tendonitis, tennis elbow

- Arthritis, gout, rheumatism

Digestive

- Improvement of metabolism
- Digestive and carminative
- Eases constipation

Invigorating

- Improves memory
- Drives energy levels up
- Reduces lethargy
- Encourages the flow of breast milk

Respiratory

- If it gets slimy and sticky Holy Basil can help.
- Catarrh, bronchitis, phlegm all those delightful things

Skin

- Reduces oil and greasy complexions
- Reduces compacted redness in the skin

Balances the temperature

- Kapha is by nature cold, so is warming but can also cool in warm weather
- Reduces stress
- Calms headaches

- Stabilising to heart complaints, and reduces cholesterol
- Enhances verbal and creative expression

If in doubt, think of oils that improve kapha as *Stimulating, Energising, Drying* and being *Expressive.*

Other references to ancient usage are more widespread than you would imagine. In Queensland, Australia, the indigenous peoples use Tulsi to alleviate fevers and sickness. In Indonesia it is used in the bath as a sedative and to ease nerve pain.

In the Highlands of the Himalayas Tulsi seeds are ground up and used in a hallucinogenic blend to bring on waking visions. The blend consists of *Sugundi root, Bel fruit, Blue Lotus, Kutuka and safflower*. I don't know, but I would suggest that the Tulsi awakens the consciousness but is not the actual hallucinogenic dimension given that it would then mean it could not be sattvic.

Holy Basil Tincture

Most of the clinical trials you will see done with Tulsi are enquiries into how **the herb** performs rather than the essential oil. To monitor their results, scientists use an ethanol extraction. You may also have heard of this in natural medicine as a **tincture**. The process of how to make these is exactly the same, except in the laboratory 100% alcohol is used and it is rare we can find this commercially without a license. (Perfumers, for instance, would use ethanol, but not aromatherapists, if that makes sense).

This difference in the plant derivative is an important distinction, because for some plants, not all active constituents are able to cross through distillation into the essential oil (like the cancer fighting constituents in frankincense for instance; they are in boswellia extract but not the essential oil). I have searched long and hard to find data that would tell me if any do not cross and but that information seems not to readily exist....but we can't take that as confirmation that the oil *is* wholly intact.

Should you want to emulate the effects they are achieving from a tincture, rather than an essential oil, this is easy to do, and actually is safer to take internally. You could also make a maceration out of oil for external use, and this is lovely way to use up the autumnal resources before the plant goes dormant for the winter.

The clinical trials are almost always performed using dried leaves, but fresh leaves work just as well. I have made good ones with a mixture of both. It is possible to find 100% proof Russian Vodka, but frankly if I used that I would be bouncing off the walls, so I just get supermarket own brand and use that. It is not as strong but it does the job. If you are tea total you can also use vinegar or glycerine, which is usually found in the cake decorating aisle of the supermarket if you get stuck. Clearly glycerine is a lot nicer than vinegar but not a good plan for diabetics.

To make a basil tincture

- Take a kilner jar (Mason jar in the States?)
- Fill the jar with as much basil as you can cram in. This will enable you to measure how much plant matter you have.
- Remove it from the jar and give it a good wash.
- Now tear the leaves and drop them into the pot.
- The more you tear the more oil you will release.

Add enough fresh chopped herbs to fill the glass container. Then add enough alcohol/vinegar / glycerine to cover

- *OR*

Add 4 oz (113g) of dried herb with 1 pint (473ml) of alcohol/ vinegar/glycerine)

- Pour over the alcohol and put a lid on.
- Label with the date and leave to stand for a month.
- Keep visiting the jar, shaking it to agitate the leaves and to enjoy the excitement about the fantastic medicine you are making!

- After a month, strain the liquid into a new container. I do this by putting a coffee filter into a funnel and then pouring into a new jar.

For a maceration, simply replace alcohol for vegetable oil.

½ tsp tincture a day is a *sooper dooper medicine*. Now let's have a look at what the scientists agree this tincture will help.

Chapter 4 Twenty First Century Usage of Tulasi

Prepare yourself for three things in this chapter.

- To be astounded at the sheer variety of things this plant has been proven to do.
- Feel very sorry for rats and mice who seem to suffer terribly in the quest for health through Holy Basil
- Possibly get slightly frustrated at the quality of the pictures of the clinical data.

I struggled long and hard about whether to do them in high definition colour- all singing-all dancing, but in the end felt it was not enough to warrant you paying almost three times as much to read the book. All of the data is taken from pubmed .com and so if you put the titles into their search engine you will be able to read the reports more fully, if you should so desire.

With reference to the bunnies: (I was going to release this book at Easter but even my warped sense of humour is starting to feel that might seem a tad black! Ah what the heck...)

Because there is so much clinical data, I will give you a list of the things it has been proven to treat and then what follows is the evidence to support this.

- Adaptogen
- Analgesic
- Heals and protects against stomach ulcers
- Reduces stomach acid

- Increases gastrointestinal protective mucous
- Protects against tooth decay, periodontis and some oral bacteria
- Aids bone healing
- Reverses oxidative stress from smoking
- Increases immunity
- Combats swine flu
- Anti inflammatory
- Aids cardiac health, reduces cholesterol and promotes vascular health
- Protects the lungs
- Anti diabetic
- Protects and regenerates liver tissue
- Anti fungal
- Heals and protects the yes against cataracts
- Anti parasitic
- Protects the body against radiation damage
- Protects against skin, liver, oral and lung cancers through anti-oxidant properties
- Causes cell death in prostate cancer cells

Clinical Evidence of the Physical Effects of Holy Basil

Adaptogen

This is a word that seems to be thrown around with more gusto than rice at weddings. But what exactly does it mean? In actual fact, it is an extraordinarily important claim.

Adaptogen means it helps the body systems return back to homeostatis after stress. Homeostasis relies on a number of intricate signals in the internal mechanism of the body to achieve:

- Normalised blood sugar
- Normalised temperature
- Stabilised water content

This is rather an over arching statement so let's consider it a little more deeply.

First let's consider where the stress might come from.

We might say psychological stress where we think of the boss on your back at work or a marriage breakdown for instance, or even just trying to be too many things to too many people. We all recognise psychological stress.

Physical stress then, what might that look like? How about long periods of illness, training for a triathlon, having a newborn baby that cannot yet let you sleep, all of these are good examples and I am sure you can think of many more.

Spiritual stress? Thoughts from the top of my head: being separated from loved ones, being in a job that kills your soul, finding out you never knew the person you have married at all.

Dietary stress: eating foods washed with fertilisers and petrochemicals, treating the body like a weapon with actions pertaining to an eating disorder.

The list could go on and on couldn't it?

If you consider that the word stress is an engineering term from the 1930s meaning "how well a substance copes with pressure" you get to see how wide reaching the effects of stress might be.

Most important to remember though, is regardless of the *source* of stress, the body will react with the same physiological processes. That is to say that it doesn't matter if you stay up too late watching box sets of Scandal on TV, if you insist on gorging on McDonalds or conversely starving yourself, or if you plummet into emotional decline because your husband leaves you….the body always kicks in the same stress response.

We call this the HPA axis, and it is covered in far more detail in <u>The Professional Stress Solution</u>, but HPA stands for

- **H**ypothalamus
- **P**ituitary

- **A**drenals

Together these three trigger a range of hormones to help the body fend off dangers it perceives. They keep on secreting and keep on secreting until the body has very little reserve left at all.

- Metabolism goes off kilter
- Immunity drops
- Sleep gets its coat and leaves
- Concentration is shot
- And life expectancy is shortened

What is fascinating is that adaptogens are able to switch off this cataclysmic health decline and reset the body to "Factory Settings".

So how do we know this?

Well the thanks must really go to two Russian scientists Dr Nikoli Lazarev (and then Dr Israel Brekman. Lazarev was a renowned pharmacologist and physician who was sequestered to research into how the Russian Army might be able to improve performance on the battle field. His research enabled him to test many products that improve performance and stamina and reduce fatigue. The soldiers, unwitting guinea pigs really, were administered with all manner of psychedelic cocktails from methamphetamines to crack cocaine. Sure enough a super battalion started to emerge, but Lazarev became more and more concerned about the side effects showing in soldiers coming home from the front. It soon became clear these products were far too powerful for long term usage. So he turned his attentions to plants.

Over time he was able to identify that a small number of plants were able to do the same as the drugs had, but in a more gentle and sustainable manner. From this, in 1947, he derived a set of guidelines as to what a plant must be to achieve the title of adaptogen.

- 1). Safety of the adaptogen's action on the organism;
- 2). A wide range of regulatory activity, but manifesting its action only against the actual challenge to the system;
- 3). Act through a nonspecific mechanism to increase the nonspecific resistance of (NSR) to harmful influences of an extremely wide spectrum of physical, chemical and biological factors causing stress;
- 4). Has a normalizing action irrespective of the direction of foregoing pathological changes.

In 1945, a young ambitious Israel Brekman was sent to work under Lazarev and he took these original guidelines and worked tirelessly to build on the database of plants which might fall under this header. Brekman furthered the research by gradually identifying which were the active components of a plant that created the adaptogenic magic.

Prolific does not even begin to describe the range of Brekmans work achieving 40 patents and 21 international patents, publishing 22 monographs and authoring literally hundreds of scientific articles.

Brekmans initial research focused on the plant Eluethro and its reputed benefits. This research and subsequent monograph about it, led to approval by the USSR for *clinical* use of Eleuthro as a stimulant.

In 1985 the Russian parliament bestowed the highest civilian honour on him, The Lenin Medal of Valiant Work as well as The Certificate of Honour.

What I find most fascinating, especially in terms of this particular book is that Lazarev's initial hunch about adaptogens came from looking at the plants used by ancient medicinal systems and indigenous medicines and noticing how they were described as "Kingly" or Elite". In China such herbs were given to soldiers before battle. In Siberia, hunters consumed them before leaving on their arduous journeys to pursue prey. Until Lazarev and Brekman commenced their joint paper in 1948, there had never been such a complete study of these plants undertaken.

It is believed that its findings were to become vital in the resurgence of the power of the Soviet States. It has been suggested that the incredible success of the space race by the Russian cosmonauts and the domination of the Olympics by their superhuman strength might possibly be attributed to adaptogenic plants, whether we will ever know if that could actually be substantiated remains to be seen.

What you will find over the coming pages are the edited highlights of literally thousands of studies into what Holy Basil might be able to achieve if it were made into a medicine. For the most part each simply takes it as read that the reader agrees that the herb *is* adaptogen without looking for research results to back that up. In some papers however, you will see that results show us certain aspects of its truth (for instance in diabetes studies it normalises blood sugar.)

More recently, studies of how Holy Basil affects the stress hormones have validated its usage even further, as it has now been proven that not only do levels of the stress hormone cortisol drop when exposed to the herb, but Holy Basil also normalises levels of epinephrine (which is what most of us know as adrenaline) as well as noradrenaline (which keeps us on danger alert) and our mood modulator serotonin.

I think it is worth elucidating here that raised levels of cortisol and low levels of serotonin are connected to depressed mood as well as poor memory and a mental fogginess.

Analgesic

Basil is one of our main pain relief oils so I am surprised there are so few investigations into why this might be. One very concise study from 2003 showed that rats were given a writhing test (Unsmiley Face!). Holy Basil affected the serotonin release, which lead the researchers to surmise that the actions occurred in the central nervous system and then in the actual nerves. I suppose we can say here, then, they suspect the extract affected not only the actual nerve pain but also the perception of it too.

I am glad to report that the rats writhing reduced and they also stopped flicking their tails in pain as much as they had been.

> Abstract ▼
>
> J Ethnopharmacol. 2003 Oct;88(2-3):293-6
>
> **Antinociceptive action of Ocimum sanctum (Tulsi) in mice: possible mechanisms involved.**
>
> Khanna N[1], Bhatia J.
>
> ⊕ Author information
>
> Abstract
>
> The alcoholic leaf extract of Ocimum sanctum (OS, Tulsi) was tested for analgesic activity in mice. In the glacial acetic acid (GAA)-induced writhing test, OS (50, 100 mg/kg, i.p.; and 50, 100, 200 mg/kg, p.o.) reduced the number of writhes. OS (50, 100 mg/kg, i.p.) also increased the tail withdrawal latency in mice. Naloxone (1 mg/kg, i.p.), an opioid antagonist, and DSP-4 (50 mg/kg, i.p.), a central noradrenaline depletor, attenuated the analgesic effect of OS in both the experimental models, whereas, PCPA (300 mg/kg, i.p.), a serotonin synthesis inhibitor, potentiated the action of OS on tail flick response in mice. The results of our study suggest that the analgesic action of OS is exerted both centrally as well as peripherally and involves an interplay between various neurotransmitter systems.
>
> PMID: 12963158 [PubMed - indexed for MEDLINE]

Gastro-Intestinal

Again, surprisingly there is little data in this area. Scientists in West Bengal, 1993, tried to assess whether tulsi could improve the damage they had done to some rats, ulcerating their intestines with aspirin. A second study was done giving the rodents tulsi extract before the aspirin was administered. Improvement was seen in the condition of the stomach ulcers in both trials. This was attributed to the way tulsi **reduces the amount of acid in the stomach**, and **also increases the volume of its protective mucous.**

Teeth

Chewing tulsi leaves is extremely common in India and evidence seems to overwhelmingly support its use as a preventative to tooth decay.

Periodontis

Peridontis is a common but very dangerous infection of the gums and bones which support your teeth. Initially presenting as bleeding gums and tooth loss it can eventually lead to heart attack or stroke. In a cross-discipline study, five separate departments from Mangalore and Karnataka in India studied the effects of tulsi on chemically induced periodontis in rats. It was found that 2% dilution in a gel could inhibit the oedema caused by the bacteria and was declared to be an effective treatment.

> **Int J Pharm Investig.** 2015 Jan-Mar;5(1):35-42. doi: 10.4103/2230-973X.147231
>
> **Evaluation of the efficacy of 2% Ocimum sanctum gel in the treatment of experimental periodontitis.**
>
> Hosadurga RR[1], Rao SN[2], Edavanputhalath R[2], Jose J[3], Rompicharla NC[3], Shakil M[4], Raju S[5].
>
> ⊕ Author information
>
> **Abstract**
> **INTRODUCTION:** One of the options for the treatment of periodontitis is local drug delivery systems (LDD). Tulsi (Ocimum sanctum), a traditional herb, has many uses in medicine. It could be a suitable agent as LDD for the treatment of periodontitis.
>
> **AIM:** The aim was to formulate, evaluate the anti-inflammatory activity, assess duration of the action and the efficacy of 2% tulsi (O. sanctum) gel in the treatment of experimental periodontitis in Wistar Albino rat model.
>
> **SETTINGS AND DESIGN:** Thirty six Wistar albino rats were randomly assigned to 3 groups. Periodontitis was induced using ligature model. Group 1-control; Group 2-Plain gel and Group 3-2% tulsi (O. sanctum) gel.
>
> **MATERIALS AND METHODS:** 2% tulsi (O. sanctum) gel were prepared. The anti-inflammatory activity and duration of action were assessed. Silk ligature 5-0 was used to induce periodontitis. Gingival index (GI) and probing pocket depth were measured. Treatment was done. The rats were sacrificed. Morphometric analysis was done using Stereomicroscope and ImageJ software.
>
> **STATISTICAL ANALYSIS USED:** ANOVA followed by Bonferroni's test, Wilcoxon's test for intergroup comparison, Mann-Whitney test for P value computation was used. The observations are mean ± standard deviation and standard error of the mean. $P < 0.01$ as compared to control was considered as statistically significant.
>
> **RESULTS:** 2% tulsi (O. sanctum) gel showed 33.66% inhibition of edema and peak activity was noted at 24 h. There was statistically significant change in the GI and probing pocket depth. Morphometric analysis did not show any significant difference between groups. No toxic effects were seen on oral administration of 2000 mg/kg of Tulsi extract.
>
> **CONCLUSIONS:** 2% tulsi (O. sanctum) gel was effective in the treatment of experimental periodontitis.

Teeth again....

This time Sacred Basil is tested in the field of endodontics, which is the dental pulp of your teeth. (Who knew there were so many types of dentists...?! All of them seem like pretty gruesome jobs to me!)

This time the study pertains to bacteria which can affect the teeth and gums. It was found that *Ocimum sanctum* was affective against streptococcus mutans at 3% dilution. This delightful bacterium inhabits the oral cavity and is one of the main protagonists of tooth decay and cavities.

> **Abstract**
>
> Eur J Dent. 2014 Apr;8(2):172-7. doi: 10.4103/1305-7456.130591.
>
> **The antimicrobial activity of Azadirachta indica, Mimusops elengi, Tinospora cardifolia, Ocimum sanctum and 2% chlorhexidine gluconate on common endodontic pathogens: An in vitro study.**
>
> Mistry KS[1], Sanghvi Z[2], Parmar G[3], Shah S[4].
>
> Author information
> [1]Department of Conservative Dentistry and Endodontics, Faculty of Dental Science, Dharamsinh Desai University, Nadiad, Gujarat, India.
> [2]Department of Conservative Dentistry and Endodontics, Ahmedabad Dental College and Hospital, Ahmedabad, Gujarat, India.
> [3]Department of Conservative Dentistry and Endodontics, Government Dental College and Hospital, Ahmedabad, Gujarat, India.
> [4]Department of Pharmacology, Sardar Patel College of Pharmacy, Anand, Gujarat, India.
>
> **Abstract**
> **OBJECTIVE:** To check the antimicrobial activity of Azadirachta indica (Neem), Ocimum sanctum (Tulsi), Mimusops elengi (Bakul), Tinospora cardifolia (Giloy) and Chlorhexidine Gluconate (CHX) on common endodontic pathogens like Streptococcus mutans, Enterococcus faecalis and staphylococcus aureus.
> **MATERIALS AND METHODS:** The agar diffusion test was used to check the antimicrobial activity of the Methanolic extracts of the medicinal plants along with CHX. Six different concentrations of the tested agents were used for the study. The values of Zone of Inhibition were tabulated according to the concentration of the tested agent and data was statistically analyzed using ANOVA and Bonferroni post- hoc tests. The Minimum Inhibitory Concentration (MIC) and Minimum Bactericidal Concentrations (MBC) values were also recorded.
> **RESULTS:** All the plants extracts showed considerable antimicrobial activity against endodontic pathogens. At 3mg. concentration, O.sanctum was the most effective against S. mutans, M. elengi showed highest zone of inhibition against E.faecalis, whereas CHX was the most effective agent against S.aureus. CHX was also the most consistent of all the medicaments testes, showing inhibitory effect against all the tree pathogens at all the selected concentrations.
> **CONCLUSIONS:** The Methanolic extract of A.Indica, O.sanctum, M. Elengi, T.cardifolia and Chlorhexidine Gluconate has considerable antimicrobial activity against S. mutans, E. faecalis and S. aureus.

A further study wanted to find the absolutely best killer dosage to whack the streptococcus mutans for good. The superhero dose was found to be 4% dilution.

> **Abstract**
>
> Indian J Dent Res. 2010 Jul-Sep;21(3):357-9. doi: 10.4103/0970-9290.70800.
>
> **Evaluation of the antimicrobial activity of various concentrations of Tulsi (Ocimum sanctum) extract against Streptococcus mutans: an in vitro study.**
>
> Agarwal P[1], Nagesh L, Murlikrishnan.
>
> Author information
>
> **Abstract**
> **AIM:** To determine if Tulsi (Ocimum sanctum) extract has an antimicrobial activity against Streptococcus mutans and to determine which concentration of Tulsi (Ocimum sanctum) extract among the 15 concentrations investigated has the maximum antimicrobial activity.
> **SETTING AND DESIGN:** Experimental design, in vitro study. Lab setting.
> **MATERIALS AND METHODS:** Ethanolic extract of Tulsi was prepared by the cold extraction method. The extract was then diluted with an inert solvent, dimethyl formamide, to obtain 15 different concentrations (0.5%, 1%, 1.5%, 2%, 2.5%, 3%, 3.5%, 4%, 4.5%, 5%, 6%, 7% 8%, 9%, 10%) of the extract. 0.2% chlorhexidine was used as a positive control and dimethyl formamide was used as a negative control. The extract, along with the controls, was then subjected to microbiological investigation to determine which concentration among the 15 different concentrations of the extract gave a wider inhibition zone against Streptococcus mutans. The zones of inhibition were measured in millimeters using a vernier caliper.
> **RESULTS:** At the 4% concentration of Tulsi extract, a zone of inhibition of 22 mm was obtained. This was the widest zone of inhibition observed among all the 15 different concentrations of Tulsi that were investigated.
> **CONCLUSION:** Tulsi extract demonstrated an antimicrobial property against Streptococcus mutans.
>
> PMID: 20930344 [PubMed - indexed for MEDLINE] Free full text

Root canal

A 2013 study monitored the effects on Holy basil on *Enterococcus faecalis* and its role in the root canal. In fact, this little nasty lives in the gastrointestinal tract and is responsible for some terrible illnesses especially passed along in the hospital environment.

> **Abstract**
>
> J Conserv Dent. 2013 Sep;16(5):454-7. doi: 10.4103/0972-0707.117507
>
> **Antibacterial efficacy of Mangifera indica L. kernel and Ocimum sanctum L. leaves against Enterococcus faecalis dentinal biofilm.**
>
> Subbiya A[1], Mahalakshmi K, Pushpangadan S, Padmavathy K, Vivekanandan P, Sukumaran VG.
>
> Author information
>
> **Abstract**
> **INTRODUCTION:** The Enterococcus faecalis biofilm in the root canal makes it difficult to be eradicated by the conventional irrigants with no toxicity to the tissues. Hence, plant products with least side effects are explored for their use as irrigants in the root canal therapy.
> **AIM:** To evaluate and compare the antibacterial efficacy of Mangifera indica L. kernel (mango kernel) and Ocimum sanctum L. leaves (tulsi) extracts with conventional irrigants (5% sodium hypochlorite (NaOCl) and 2% chlorhexidine) against E. faecalis dentinal biofilm.
> **MATERIALS AND METHODS:** Agar diffusion and broth microdilution assay was performed with the herbal extracts and conventional irrigants (2% chlorhexidine and 5% NaOCl) against E. faecalis planktonic cells. The assay was extended onto 3 week E. faecalis dentinal biofilm.
> **RESULTS:** Significant reduction of colony forming units (CFU)/mL was observed for the herbal groups and the antibacterial activity of the herbal groups was at par with 5% NaOCl.
> **CONCLUSIONS:** The antibacterial activity of these herbal extracts is found to be comparable with that of conventional irrigants both on the biofilm and planktonic counterparts.
>
> **KEYWORDS:** Antibacterial activity; Enterococcus faecalis biofilm; mango kernel; root canal; tulsi leaves
>
> PMID: 24082577 [PubMed] PMCID: PMC3778630   Free PMC Article

Here the effects of two different strains of tulsi were tested (along with mango kernel). Again, we see preparations of dry leaves mixed and extracted (not essential oils) and placed into petri dishes with *Enterococcus faecalis*. While the mango kernel was the most effective in eradicating the bug, all three extracts (Mango kernel and two tulsis) were found to be as effective as the conventional method of irrigating the canal with chlorohexadine and sodium hypochlorite.

Bone Healing

There was a beautifully sensitive piece written by The Department of Oral and Maxillofacial Surgery, from St Georges in Uttar Pradesh about how useful plant extracts could be to speed healing of particularly difficult fractures of the jaw.

It is easy to forget that bone is a living tissue. It is entirely reliant on hormones, nutrition and vascular health to function well. The high nutritional content of tulsi makes it a perfect aid to skeletal healing. It was found that patients who had been administered powdered tulsi mixed with 80% alcohol had to have their jaw immobilised for a far shorter time than both the placebo group, and those treated with a member of the grape family *Cissus quadrangularis*. Each test subject was given a teaspoon of the treatment 2.5g every six hours of tulsi and 3.5g every eight hours of Cissus.

Those treated with cissus however, were able to regain strength in their bite far more quickly than those treated with basil. That is to say Holy basil speeds healing but, in this case at least, cissus was the means to making the jaw bone become stronger.

> Abstract ▾
>
> Natl J Maxillofac Surg. 2014 Jan;5(1):35-8. doi: 10.4103/0975-5950.140167.
> **Herbal remedies for mandibular fracture healing.**
> Mohammad S[1], Pal US[1], Pradhan R[1], Singh N[1].
>
> Author information
> [1]Department of Oral and Maxillofacial Surgery, King George's Medical University, Lucknow, Uttar Pradesh, India.
>
> Abstract
> **PURPOSE:** When a bone is fractured it is usually necessary to employ a mechanical means to reduce and maintain the fragments in position. However, healing of the fracture is governed by biological principles, with which the mechanical measures must be coordinated to the end, such that a satisfactory bony union and restoration of form and function are obtained. We have studied the effect of Cissus quadrangularis (Harjor) and Ocimum sanctum (Tulsi), in the healing of mandibular fractures.
> **MATERIALS AND METHODS:** A total of 29 cases having a fracture in the body of the mandible were included in the study and divided into three groups. Groups A and B were treated with Ocimum sanctum and Cissus quadrangularis, respectively, and fracture healing was assessed with biochemical markers and the bite force. Group C was the control group.
> **RESULTS:** The period of immobilization was the lowest in the Group A followed by Group B. A significant increase in alkaline phosphatase and serum calcium was seen in Group B. The tensile strength in terms of the biting force was the maximum in cases of Group B.
> **CONCLUSION:** We conclude that Cissus quadrangularis and Ocimum sanctum help in fracture healing, and use of such traditional drugs will be a breakthrough in the management and early mobilization of facial fractures.
>
> **KEYWORDS:** Alkaline phosphatase; Cissus quadrangularis; Ocimum sanctum
>
> PMID: 25298715 [PubMed]   PMCID: PMC4178353   Free PMC Article

Oxidative Stress from Smoking

A poor chicken embryo (c9 days old) was used to try to help people who insist on trying to kill themselves with cigarettes. Nicotine was administered to the embryo and was seen to go black. A variety of herbals were assessed with neem performing the best in recovering the oxidative stress to the cells (70% improvement) followed by tulsi which engineered a 65% improvement in the condition of the cells. The herbs were administered in powdered form. 250g of tulsi, the same was used of neem with 5ml of distilled water from a pipette. It was found the best possible ratio of improvement was achieved with 3:1 ratio Neem: tulsi

Immune Response

Mickey's mousey mates get a rest in the next trial and amazingly we have data from actual humans! 27 healthy chaps and chappesses were given capsules of tulsi to measure the difference it made on their immune systems, in comparison to a placebo group. After four weeks they were found to have increased levels of helper cells and natural killer cells clearly demonstrating an improved immune system.

> Abstract
>
> J Ethnopharmacol. 2011 Jul 14;136(3):452-6. doi: 10.1016/j.jep.2011.05.012. Epub 2011 May 17.
>
> **Double-blinded randomized controlled trial for immunomodulatory effects of Tulsi (Ocimum sanctum Linn.) leaf extract on healthy volunteers.**
>
> Mondal S[1], Varma S, Bamola VD, Naik SN, Mirdha BR, Padhi MM, Mehta N, Mahapatra SC.
>
> Author information
>
> Abstract
>
> **ETHNOPHARMACOLOGICAL RELEVANCE:** Tulsi (Ocimum sanctum Linn.) is considered as a sacred herb and traditionally it is believed that consumption of Tulsi leaf on empty stomach increases immunity. Experimental studies have shown that alcoholic extract of Tulsi modulates immunity.
>
> **MATERIALS AND METHODS:** The present study was designed to evaluate the immunomodulatory effects of ethanolic extract of Tulsi leaves through a double-blinded randomized controlled cross-over trial on healthy volunteers. Three hundred milligrams capsules of ethanolic extracts of leaves of Tulsi or placebo were administered to 24 healthy volunteers on empty stomach and the results of 22 subjects who completed the study were analyzed. The primary objective was to study the levels of Th1 and Th2 cytokines (interferon-γ and interleukin-4) during both pre and post intervention period in blood culture supernatants following stimulation with lipopolysaccharide and phytohaemagglutinin. Other immunological parameters such as T-helper and T-cytotoxic cells, B-cells and NK-cells also were analyzed using Flowcytometry.
>
> **RESULTS:** Statistically significant increase in the levels of IFN-γ (p=0.039), IL-4 (p=0.001) and percentages of T-helper cells (p=0.001) and NK-cells (p=0.017) were observed after 4 weeks in the Tulsi extract intervention group in contrast to the placebo group.
>
> **CONCLUSIONS:** These observations clearly ascertain the immunomodulatory role of Tulsi leaves extract on healthy volunteers.
>
> Copyright © 2011 Elsevier Ireland Ltd. All rights reserved.
>
> PMID: 21616917 [PubMed - indexed for MEDLINE]

Swine Flu

> Indian J Pharm Sci. 2014 Jan;76(1):10-8.
>
> **In Silico Analysis to Compare the Effectiveness of Assorted Drugs Prescribed for Swine flu in Diverse Medicine Systems.**
>
> Raja K[1], Prabahar A[1], Selvakumar S[1], Raja TK[2].
>
> Author information
>
> **Abstract**
>
> The genome of the virus H1N1 2009 consists of eight segments but maximum number of mutations occurs at segments 1 and 4, coding for PB2 subunit of hemagglutinin. Comparatively less number of mutations occur at segment 6, coding for neuraminidase. Two antiviral drugs, oseltamivir and zanamivir are commonly prescribed for treating H1N1 infection. Alternate medical systems do compete equally; andrographolide in Siddha and gelsemine in Homeopathy. Recent studies confirm the efficacy of eugenol from Tulsi and vitamins C and E against H1N1. As the protein structures are unavailable, we modeled them using Modeller by identifying suitable templates, 1RUY and 3BEQ, for hemagglutinin and neuraminidase, respectively. Prior to docking simulations using AutoDock, the drug likeness properties of the ligands were screened using in silico techniques. Docking results showed interaction between the proteins individually into selected ligands, except for gelsemine and vitamin E no interactions were shown. The best docking simulation was reported by vitamin C interacting through six hydrogen bonds into proteins hemagglutinin and neuraminidase with binding energies -4.28 and -4.56 kcal/mol, respectively. Furthermore, vitamin C showed hydrophobic interactions with both proteins, two bonds with Arg119, Glu120 of HA, and one bond with Arg74 of NA. In silico docking studies thus recommend vitamin C to be more effective against H1N1.
>
> **KEYWORDS:** H1N1; Swine flu; Tamiflu; hemagglutinin; neuraminidase; vitamin C
>
> PMID: 24790734 [PubMed] PMCID: PMC4007250 Free PMC Article

This study by Tamil Nadu University confirms that there are two orthodox vaccinations in circulation. Tamiflu (Oseltamivir) and the lesser known Relenza (Zanamivir); Relenza is described as being the most effective. Later in the article it states:

"Ayurveda, another ancient medicine system of India, reports the best form of herbal remedies for swine flu. This corroborates with a natural product called eugenol from Tulsi *(Holy Basil) for curing swine flu. Eugenol is an essential oil present in high concentration in* Tulsi, *which has both antiviral and anti-inflammatory properties."*

Incidentally don't forget that euganol is also found in even higher concentration in clove oil.

Anti-inflammatory Action

> **Abstract**
>
> J Ethnopharmacol. 2014 May 28;154(1):148-55. doi: 10.1016/j.jep.2014.03.049. Epub 2014 Apr 13.
>
> **Ocimum sanctum leaf extracts attenuate human monocytic (THP-1) cell activation.**
>
> Choudhury SS[1], Bashyam L[2], Manthapuram N[2], Bitla P[2], Kolipara P[3], Tetali SD[4].
>
> Author information
>
> **Abstract**
>
> **ETHNOPHARMACOLOGICAL RELEVANCE:** Ocimum sanctum (OS), commonly known as Holy basil/Tulsi, has been traditionally used to treat cardiovascular diseases (CVD) and manage general cardiac health. The present study is designed to evaluate the antiinflammatory effect of O. sanctum and its phenolic compound and eugenol (EUG) in human monocytic (THP-1) cells and validate its traditional use for treating cardiovascular diseases.
>
> **MATERIALS AND METHODS:** The phytochemical analysis of alcoholic and water extracts of OS-dry leaves (OSAE and OSWE) was done using LC-QTOF-MS. A phenolic compound, EUG was quantified in both OSAE and OSWE by an LC-MS technique using a mass hunter work station software quantitative analysis system. The effect of both OSAE, OSWE, pure compound EUG and positive control imatinib (IMT) was investigated in THP-1 cells by studying the following markers: lipopolysaccharide (LPS) induced tumor necrosis factor alpha (TNF-α) secretion by ELISA, gene expression of inflammatory markers (TNF-α, IL-6, MIP-1α and MCP-1) by real time PCR and translocation of nuclear factor kappa B (NF-κB) by confocal microscopy. Furthermore, the effect of the extracts, EUG and IMT, was studied on phorbol-12-myristate-13-acetate (PMA) induced monocyte to macrophage differentiation and gene expression of CD14, TLR2 and TLR4.
>
> **RESULTS:** The LC-MS analysis of OSAE and OSWE revealed the presence of several bioactive compounds including eugenol. Quantitative analysis revealed that OSAE and OSWE had EUG of 12 ng/mgdwt and 19 ng/mgdwt respectively. OSAE, OSWE (1 mg dwt/mL) pure compound EUG (60 μg/mL) and positive control IMT (20 μg/mL) showed marked inhibition on LPS induced TNF-α secretion by THP-1 cells. At the selected concentration, the plant extracts, EUG and IMT inhibited gene expression of cytokines and chemokines (IL-6, TNF-α, MIP-1α, MCP-1) and translocation of NF-κB-p65 to the nuclei. In addition, they showed significant inhibition on PMA induced monocyte to macrophage differentiation and the gene expression of CD14, TLR2 and TLR4 markers.
>
> **CONCLUSION:** The result of the present study validated traditional use of Ocimum sanctum for treating cardiovascular disease for the first time by testing antiinflammatory activity of Ocimum sanctum in acute inflammatory model, LPS induced THP-1 cells. The plant extracts showed significant antiinflammatory activity, however, further to be evaluated using chronic inflammatory animal models like diabetic or apolipoprotein E-deficient mice to make it evidence based medicine. The phenolic compound eugenol (60 μg/mL) showed significant antiinflammatory activity. However the amount of eugenol present in 1mg of OSAE and OSWE (12 ng/mg dwt and 19 ng/mg dwt respectively) used for cell based assays was very low. It suggests that several other metabolites along with eugenol are responsible for the efficacy of the extracts.
>
> Copyright © 2014 Elsevier Ireland Ltd. All rights reserved.

Ok, so this is a fascinating article but you will need your physiology head well and truly screwed on to understand what it says. The first bit is clear, scientists in Hyderabad wanted to confirm or deny alternative medicine's claims that Tulsi could help to manage cardio vascular diseases and also help cardiac health in general. Their outcome was to discover that, yes, it could.

They made water and alcohol extracts from dried herbs to do their tests (not essential oils). Their tests showed that **compounds inhibited the expression of TNF alpha**

expression. This horrid little blighter will be familiar to those of you have read my *Aromatherapy Bronchitis Treatment* book as **one of the main protagonists of inflammation in the body**. Sacred Basil also prevented the creation of cytokines and chemokines, as well as macrophages, all of which are responsible for triggering immune responses that cause inflammation.

This report is a nice one to read because it tells us where they want to take that finding next. We know they are interested in exploring the heart, but they feel this might have relevance to diabetes too, and so will escalate the research onto the poor old mice to see what happens.

Interestingly too, here they suspect the action may not be entirely down to euganol because the levels seems so small and so perhaps there are other compounds not yet identified which might be doing the job.

Stress

Poor old rabbits are suffering in the name of Holy Basil research here.

Little white bunnies had hypoxic anaemia induced by injection of sodium nitrite to raise their physiological stress responses. It is a short paper but the gist is that thankfully they chilled out. Their cardio-respiratory changes improved and their blood sugar levelled. The scientists felt this was because of the anti-oxidant properties contained within their fresh crunchy tulsi leaves.

Blissed out basil bunnies...!

Bless their little cottonball bums.

But if we look at it with a bit more of a serious head on. Cardio respiratory processes slowed, blood sugars levelled....

Hello adaptogen evidence.

> Abstract ▾
>
> Methods Find Exp Clin Pharmacol. 2007 Jul-Aug;29(6):411-6.
>
> **Antistressor activity of Ocimum sanctum (Tulsi) against experimentally induced oxidative stress in rabbits.**
>
> Jyoti S[1], Satendra S, Sushma S, Anjana T, Shashi S.
>
> ⊕ Author information
>
> Abstract
>
> Fresh leaves of Ocimum sanctum (O. sanctum) were evaluated for antistress activity against experimentally induced oxidative stress in albino rabbits. Animals of the test group received supplementation of 2 g fresh leaves of O. sanctum per rabbit for 30 days. Anemic hypoxia was induced chemically by injecting the rabbits with 15 mg sodium nitrite per 100 g body weight intraperitoneally. Results indicated that O. sanctum administration blunted the changes in cardiorespiratory (BP, HR, RR) parameters in response to stress. A significant (p < 0.01) decrease in blood sugar level was observed after 30 days of dietary supplementation of O. sanctum leaves. Significant increase (p < 0.05) in the levels of enzymatic (superoxide dismutase) and nonenzymatic (reduced glutathione) antioxidants was observed in the test group after the treatment with O. sanctum. Oxidative stress led to a lesser depletion of reduced glutathione (26.80%) and plasma superoxide dismutase (23.04%) in O. sanctum-treated rabbits. The results of this study suggest that the potential antistressor activity of O. sanctum is partly attributable to its antioxidant properties.
>
> PMID: 17922070 [PubMed - indexed for MEDLINE]

Lung Protection

Right, now, after feeding the next bit of research I feel as if I need to go back to my old home town to do some food shopping. In the West Midlands there is a large Asian community and my daughter and I would visit every school holidays to coo at the beautiful sari fabrics and feast on the gastro-diversity of ingredients available. Oh and to stock up on rose water from the Indian supermarkets too!

It galls me to think of the racks of tulsi all readily laid out in comparison to wealth of delicious local products here, especially when I see what supplementing with tulsi may be able to do for my lungs. In this particular study, rather than using Tulsi extract, essential oils are used.

Here the idea was to see how using tulsi and clove oils might be able to clean the lungs of the delightful bacteria *kiebsiella pneumonia*. This is a very dangerous illness for anyone with a weakened immune system, but in particular sufferers of COPD and also diabetes. Infections leading to pneumonia and broncho-pneumonia can boast mortality rates as high as 50%. The clove oil was able to clean the lungs of the bacteria after only short term usage. By contrast, even though the tulsi did just as effective job, it was slower. The supplementation by tulsi was effective after longer term usage.

I love a good succinct conclusion to a report. This one says:

"Dietary supplementation with tulsi and clove oils protects against bacterial colonization of the lungs."

I can see this part of the book unleashing all hell with the ingestion/not ingest argument. Tulsi is an extremely strong oil, ingest a tincture or oral supplement, but **not the**

essential oil please.

> Abstract
>
> J Microbiol Immunol Infect. 2009 Apr;42(2):107-13.
>
> **Induction of resistance to respiratory tract infection with Klebsiella pneumoniae in mice fed on a diet supplemented with tulsi (Ocimum sanctum) and clove (Syzgium aromaticum) oils.**
>
> Saini A[1], Sharma S, Chhibber S.
>
> Author information
>
> Abstract
>
> **BACKGROUND AND PURPOSE:** The impact of diet and specific food groups on respiratory tract infections has been widely recognized in recent years. This study was conducted to study the effect of tulsi (Ocimum sanctum) oil and clove (Syzgium aromaticum) oil on the susceptibility of experimental mice to respiratory tract infection.
>
> **METHODS:** The effect of 2 different regimens of short-term (15 days) and long-term (30 days) feeding with tulsi oil and clove oil on the course of Klebsiella pneumoniae American Type Culture Collection 43816 infection in the lungs of mice was analyzed. The operative mechanisms of lipid peroxidation/nitrite production were studied by estimating their levels in bronchoalveolar lavage fluid (BALF). Bacterial colonization, malondialdehyde (MDA) and nitrite production in BALF, and tumor necrosis factor-alpha level in serum were assessed.
>
> **RESULTS:** The results showed that there was a significant decrease in bacterial colonization after short-term feeding with clove oil compared with the controls (p < 0.05). For tulsi oil-fed mice, the decrease in bacterial load was significant with long-term feeding (p < 0.01). The maximum decrease in MDA levels and increase in nitrite levels were noted with long-term feeding.
>
> **CONCLUSION:** Dietary supplementation with tulsi and clove oils protects against bacterial colonization of the lungs.
>
> PMID: 19597641 [PubMed - indexed for MEDLINE]

Anti-diabetic

I have a particular hatred for the disease of diabetes and so I always leap on research that might show us a way out of this disastrous health decline.

The first paper I'll cite is from 2004 and here we have white rabbits coming out of the hat again. Forty of them, in fact. These were quite happy hoppers though, I think, because their job was just to munch on Holy Basil leaves for 30 days. The abstract you can see on the page is quite reserved in its findings, but the actual results of how this affected their blood sugar are astounding.

The blood sugar was found to have dropped by a whacking 26% in subjects, and the blood anti-oxidant glutathione had increased by 50.14% in comparison to readings they had taken on the first day of the trial.

> Abstract
>
> Indian J Clin Biochem. 2004 Jul;19(2):152-5. doi: 10.1007/BF02894276
>
> **Evaluation of hypoglycemic and antioxidant effect of Ocimum sanctum.**
>
> Sethi J[1], Sood S, Seth S, Talwar A.
>
> Author information
>
> Abstract
>
> Ocimum sanctum leaves have been traditionally used in treatment of diabetes mellitus. Dietary supplementation of fresh tulsi leaves in a dose of 2 gm/kg BW for 30 days led to significant lowering of blood glucose levels in test group. Intake of Ocimum sanctum also led to significant increase in levels of superoxide dismutase, reduced glutathione and total thiols, but marked reduction in peroxiodised lipid levels as compared to untreated control group. The leaves were found to possess both superoxide and hydroxyl free radical scavenging action. The present observations establish the efficacy of Ocimum sanctum leaves in lowering blood glucose levels and antioxidant property appears to be predominantly responsible for hypoglycemic effect.
>
> KEYWORDS: Ocimum sanctum; antioxidant; free radical scavenger; hypoglycemic effect
>
> PMID: 23105475 [PubMed] PMCID: PMC3454204 Free PMC Article

In the second study we have rats from 2006. The poor things had various diabetic changes induced and were left alone for a month until their eyes showed signs of retinopathy. They were then treated with Holy Basil in conjunction with vitamin E. After 16 weeks all aspects of the diabetes were showing improvements, including the levels of sugar in blood plasma, but remarkably the retinopathy was receding and they were beginning to regain some degree of sight.

> **Abstract**
>
> Indian J Clin Biochem. 2006 Sep 21(2) 181-8. doi: 10.1007/BF02912930
>
> **Effect ofOcimum sanctum (Tulsi) and vitamin E on biochemical parameters and retinopathy in streptozotocin induced diabetic rats.**
>
> Halim EM[1], Mukhopadhyay AK.
>
> Author information
>
> Abstract
> This study was carried out to see the effect of the aqueous extract ofOcitum sanctum Linn (Tulsi) with Vitamin E on biochemical parameters and retinopathy in the streptozotocin-induced diabetic albino male rats. Adult albino male rats weighing 150-200 gm were made diabetic by intraperitoneal injection of streptozotocin in the dose 60 mg/kg in citrate buffer (pH 6.3). The diabetic animals were left for one month to develop retinopathy. Biochemical parameters like plasma glucose, oral glucose tolerance and glycosylated hemoglobin HbA(1c), were measured along with lipid profile, and enzymes like glutathione peroxidase (GPX), lipid peroxidase (LPO), superoxide dismutase (SOD), catalase (CAT) and glutathione-S-transferase (GST) in normal, untreated diabetic rats and diabetic rats treated withOcimum sanctum L extracts and vitamin E. Fluorescein angiography test was done for assessing retinopathy. Results on biochemical parameters were analyzed statistically by using ANOVA followed by Dunnet's 't-test. A p-value of <0.05 was considered as significant. Evaluation of biochemical profile in treated groups showed statistically significant reduction in plasma levels of glucose, HbA(1c), lipid profile and LPO, and elevation of GPX, SOD, CAT and GST. Treatment of the diabetic animals withOcimum sanctum and Vitamin E, alone and in combination for 16 weeks showed reversal of most of the parameters studied including plasma glucose levels. Angiography showed improvement in retinal changes following combined antidiabetic treatment.
>
> **KEYWORDS:** Antioxidants; Diabetes mellitus; Diabetic retinopathy; Lipid peroxidation; Ocimum sanctum; Vitamin E
>
> PMID: 23105641 [PubMed] PMCID: PMC3453971   Free PMC Article

This 2006 study jointly run by the School of Biomedical Sciences, University of Ulster and a biomedical research group from Bangladesh was remarkable because it took the already known data that tulsi helps diabetes and tried to explain why that might be. It cleverly took dried leaves and extracted them with alcohol and then found a way to partition the various constituents and watch each of their actions in turn. They were able to ascertain that tulsi extract was able to reduce the amounts of blood sugar whilst increasing blood plasma (so the ratio became smaller and less troublesome). More importantly, here we have an assertion that it is not only rats...**this works in humans too.**

> **Abstract**
>
> J Endocrinol. 2006 Apr;189(1):127-36.
>
> **Ocimum sanctum leaf extracts stimulate insulin secretion from perfused pancreas, isolated islets and clonal pancreatic beta-cells.**
>
> Hannan JM, Marenah L, Ali L, Rokeya B, Flatt PR, Abdel-Wahab YH.
>
> Author information
>
> **Abstract**
>
> Ocimum sanctum leaves have previously been reported to reduce blood glucose when administered to rats and humans with diabetes. In the present study, the effects of ethanol extract and five partition fractions of O. sanctum leaves were studied on insulin secretion together with an evaluation of their mechanisms of action. The ethanol extract and each of the aqueous, butanol and ethylacetate fractions stimulated insulin secretion from perfused rat pancreas, isolated rat islets and a clonal rat beta-cell line in a concentration-dependent manner. The stimulatory effects of ethanol extract and each of these partition fractions were potentiated by glucose, isobutylmethylxanthine, tolbutamide and a depolarizing concentration of KCl. Inhibition of the secretory effect was observed with diazoxide, verapamil and Ca2+ removal. In contrast, the stimulatory effects of the chloroform and hexane partition fractions were associated with decreased cell viability and were unaltered by diazoxide and verapamil. The ethanol extract and the five fractions increased intracellular Ca2+ in clonal BRIN-BD11 cells, being partly attenuated by the addition of verapamil. These findings indicated that constituents of O. sanctum leaf extracts have stimulatory effects on physiological pathways of insulin secretion which may underlie its reported antidiabetic action.
>
> PMID: 16614387 [PubMed - indexed for MEDLINE] Free full text

Liver Protection

Researchers at Mahatma Gandhi Medical College and Research Institute in Ponticherry in India, tested the effects of *Ocimum sanctum* and silymarin (active constituent found in Milk Thistle) on albino rats who had had their livers hurt by paracetamol. Together they bought about significant protection to the liver. What's more as well as the reduction bought about in fatty cell growth and congestion, regeneration of the liver had begun to take place.

> Abstract ▾   Send to: ▾
>
> Pharmacognosy Res. 2011 Jan;3(1):13-8. doi: 10.4103/0974-8490.79110.
>
> **Hepatoprotective activity of Ocimum sanctum alcoholic leaf extract against paracetamol-induced liver damage in Albino rats.**
>
> Lahon K, Das S.
>
> ⊖ Author information
>
> [1]Department of Pharmacology, Mahatma Gandhi Medical College and Research Institute, Pondicherry, India.
>
> Abstract
>
> **BACKGROUND:** There is a lack of reliable hepatoprotective drugs in modern medicine to prevent and treat drug-induced liver damage. Leaves of Sacred/Holy Basil, i.e. Green Tulsi (Ocimum sanctum), belonging to family Lamiaceae are used traditionally for their hepatoprotective effect. We wanted to evaluate the hepatoprotective activity of Ocimum sanctum and observe whether synergistic hepatoprotection exists with silymarin.
>
> **MATERIALS AND METHODS:** Albino rats (150-200 g) were divided into five groups. Groups A and B were normal and experimental controls, respectively. Groups C, D and E received the alcoholic extract of Ocimum Sanctum leaves (OSE) 200 mg/kg BW/day, silymarin 100 mg/kg BW/day and OSE 100 mg/kg BW/day + silymarin 50 mg/kg BW/day p.o., respectively, for 10 days. Hepatotoxicity was induced in Groups B, C, D and E on the eighth day with paracetamol 2 g/kg BW/day. The hepatoprotective effect was evaluated by performing an assay of the serum proteins, albumin globulin ratio, alkaline phosphatase, transaminases and liver histopathology. The assay results were presented as mean and standard error of mean (SEM) for each group. The study group was compared with the control group by one-way ANOVA, followed by Bonferoni's test. A P-value of <0.01 was considered significant.
>
> **RESULTS:** In groups C, D and E, liver enzymes and albumin globulin ratio were significantly (P < 0.01) closer to normal than in group B. Reduction in sinusoidal congestion, cloudy swelling and fatty changes and regenerative areas of the liver were observed on histopathological examination in groups C, D and E, whereas group B showed only hepatic necrosis.
>
> **CONCLUSION:** The Ocimum sanctum alcoholic leaf extract shows significant hepatoprotective activity and synergism with silymarin.
>
> **KEYWORDS:** Hepatoprotective; Ocimum sanctum; hepatotoxicity; paracetamol; silymarin

Anti-Fungal

Now, can you hear my hands rubbing together in excitement? I love me a bit of antifungal data. This is stuff we base level therapists can get our teeth into; unlike diabetes and cancer treatment, anti-fungal therapy we can use in our clinics in the here and now!

Candida albacans, we all know this delightful sweetie don't we? Here we also see investigations into Candida tropicalis.

Tulsi won the competition between aloe vera and peppermint and in this particular trial we *are* actually talking about essential oils for a change, and aloe vera aqueous extract.

Active constituents doing the heavy lifting were identified as Eugenol, methyl eugenol, linalool, and 1, 8-cineole with **linalool** being the **anti-fungal superwarrior.**

Eyes

I am squirming now. I have a donor card and they can take everything from me when I go except for my eyes. Don't know why, but it seriously gives me the willies. I refused to take biology at school because there was a dissection of a sheep's eye on the syllabus. So whilst this next section is extremely important and completely fascinating, it is, to me at least, ***absolutely horrifying***.

Eyes were taken from patients aged 20-40 within 5 – 8 hours of their deaths and were treated with hydrogen peroxide. This is a major protagonist of cataracts forming on the lens of the eye.

Nope. Sorry, it's beyond me. I just can't keep reading it to describe it. Ugh, here you go, read it for yourself. Hideous.

Basically it says it worked. It stopped the formation of cataracts because of its anti-oxidant properties. Importantly it also proves that extracts can penetrate the membranes of the eye.

Wonderful…but vile.

I'll make this one as big as I can for you so I copped out so rubbishly!

> **Abstract**
>
> Phytother Res. 2009 Dec;23(12):1734-7. doi: 10.1002/ptr.2831.
>
> **Ocimum sanctum extracts attenuate hydrogen peroxide induced cytotoxic ultrastructural changes in human lens epithelial cells.**
>
> Haider N[1], Joshi S, Nag TC, Tandon R, Gupta SK.
>
> Author information
>
> Abstract
>
> Hydrogen peroxide (H2O2) is the major oxidant involved in cataract formation. The present study investigated the effect of an aqueous leaf extract of Tulsi (Ocimum sanctum) against H2O2 induced cytotoxic changes in human lens epithelial cells (HLEC). Donor eyes of the age range 20-40 years were procured within 5-8 h of death. After several washings with gentamicin (50 mL/L) and betadine (10 mL/L), clear transparent lenses (n=6 in each group) were incubated in Dulbecco's modified Eagle's medium (DMEM) alone (normal) or in DMEM containing 100 microm of H2O2 (control) or in DMEM containing both H2O2 (100 microm) and 150 microg/mL of Ocimum sanctum extract (treated) for 30 min at 37 degrees C with 5% CO2 and 95% air. Following incubation, the semi-hardened epithelium of each lens was carefully removed, fixed and processed for electron microscopic studies. Thin sections (60-70 mm) were contrasted with uranyl acetate and lead citrate and viewed under a transmission electron microscope. Normal epithelial cells showed intact, euchromatic nucleus with few small vacuoles (diameter 0.58+/-0.6 microm) in well-demarcated cytoplasm. After treatment with H2O2, they showed pyknotic nuclei with clumping of chromatin and ill-defined edges. The cytoplasm was full of vacuoles (diameter 1.61+/-0.7 microm). The overall cellular morphology was typical of dying cells. Treatment of cells with Ocimum sanctum extract protected the epithelial cells from H2O2 insult and maintained their normal architecture. The mean diameter of the vacuoles was 0.66+/-0.2 microm. The results indicate that extracts of O. sanctum have an important protective role against H2O2 injury in HLEC by maintaining the normal cellular architecture. The protection could be due to its ability to reduce H2O2 through its antioxidant property and thus reinforcing the concept that the extracts can penetrate the HLEC membrane.
>
> Copyright (c) 2009 John Wiley & Sons, Ltd.

Anti parasitic

This section could be an essay in its own right because I got so lost in the research. During a larger trial, it was found that Tulsi had strong leishmaniacal properties. Lieshmania are human protozoa that are passed as parasitcs via sand flies.

Never heard of it? Nope nor had I. But I have *seen* it a lot... I just didn't know what it was. I'll tell you why in a moment.

Interestingly this is no new kid on the block. The earliest references to the disease can be traced back to around 2000BCE from the paleotropics. Fossilised remains of the Leishmania parasite, *Paleoleishmania* have been found dating back to the cretaceous period. For those of us who are not 5 years old and named Dexter, it might be useful for me to elucidate and say that is anything from 145-66 million years ago. (And since the wee man is bound to try to read this over my shoulder at some point whilst trying to persuade me the computer would be better employed for him to watch minecraft: *No Dex, it is not a dinosaur I am afraid. It's a fly. Boring, I know.*)

In antiquity the resulting disease from a bite from the beastie was often referred to as White Leprosy or Black Fever. Today it is thought there are around 12 million sufferers worldwide in 98 countries.

So here, look at this that I wrote last year in The Aromatherapy Eczema Treatment

"Revoltingly, many of us are unwittingly playing host to unwanted visitors. There are the obvious ones like tape worm and round worm, but there can also be horrid parasites from insect bites.

If you do your job carefully, eczema flare-ups with their roots in these nasties are quite easy to spot.

Here's what you'll hear as your patient gleefully shoves some unsightly limb in your face…

"Have a look at this! Bet you've never seen anything like that before! The doctor's given me all sorts but it always seems to come back. The strange thing is, it only flares up when it's hot!" (Or may be cold on some occasions, but the key is the seasonal cycle).

From there, try to trace back how long they have had the problem. You can usually match it to a holiday. They've been attacked by some horrid fly (often from a defensive response to being stepped on in the sand) which of course they may or may not remember. When they've come home, it has been too cold for the parasite, so it has lain dormant until the sun came out. This is when you see the horrid skin lesions. Incidentally, I have also seen this happen from building sand and farm yard manure too. I actually think I picked one up years ago when I was licked by some kind of deer thing at the Safari Park and I had an open wound on my hand. The flies get in, they attack, but the patient has no idea until the insect's natural cycle recommences.

A more mundane source [of parasitic invasion] can be eating raw salad and fruit which has not been washed and of course, the one we all know: uncooked pork. Another clue which might lead you to believe there is a digestive parasite in particular is ravenous hunger. Just as the cat never stops mewling for food when she has a worm, humans respond in just the same way.

Isn't that delightful? Never mind how revolting it is, I'm absolutely certain you'll do a celebratory dance next time someone shows you their scabby hand!

I am being rather flippant about it because frankly it is vile, but the affects of parasitic infection are dreadful really. Not only could it be eczema you see, but PMS is a big one, cystitis, diarrhoea, asthma and psoriasis too.

In the words of my Advanced Aromatherapy course notes, since I have never found a better phrase: Parasites lead to an insidious breakdown of health."

Leishmaniasis, man!

Now all we have to do is try to remember the name of it…oh, and remember that Tulsi is the treatment.

The second bit, I can manage.

If you want to wade through exactly which constituent did the work, knock yourself out. You're on your own I'm afraid. I don't get paid enough for the headache all those *oxy's* are going to give me.

> Abstract ▼ Send to: ▼
>
> Chem Pharm Bull (Tokyo). 2009 Mar;57(3):245-51.
>
> **Leishmanicidal active constituents from Nepalese medicinal plant Tulsi (Ocimum sanctum L.).**
>
> Suzuki A[1], Shirota O, Mori K, Sekita S, Fuchino H, Takano A, Kuroyanagi M.
>
> Author information
>
> [1]Faculty of Life and Environmental Sciences, Prefectural University of Hiroshima, Shobara, Hiroshima 727-0023, Japan.
>
> Abstract
>
> In the course of screening leishmanicidal active compounds from Asian and South American medicinal plants, a Nepalese medicinal plant, Tulsi (Ocimum sanctum L.), showed strong activity. We therefore studied the isolation and structural elucidation of the active constituents from O. sanctum L. From the ethyl acetate soluble fraction of the plant, seven new novel neolignan derivatives were isolated along with 16 known compounds. The structures of the new compounds (1-7) were elucidated as 6-allyl-3',8-dimethoxy-flavan-3,4'-diol (1), 6-allyl-3-(4-allyl-2-methoxyphenoxy)-3',8-dimethoxyflavan-4'-ol (2), 5-allyl-3-(4-allyl-2-methoxyphenoxymethyl)-2-(4-hydroxy-3-methoxyphenyl)-7-methoxy-2,3-dihydrobenzofuran (3), 1,2-bis(4-allyl-2-methoxyphenoxy)-3-(4-hydroxy-3-methoxyphenyl)-3-methoxypropane (4), 1-(4-hydroxy-3-methoxyphenyl)-1,2,3-tris(4-allyl-2-methoxyphenoxy)propane (5), 1-allyl-4-(5-allyl-2-hydroxy-3-methoxyphenoxy)-3-(4-allyl-2-methoxyphenoxy)-5-methoxybenzene (6), and 3-(5-allyl-2-hydroxy-3-methoxyphenyl)-1-(4-hydroxy-3-methoxyphenoxy)-prop-1-ene (7) by means of (1)H-NMR, (13)C-NMR, and 2D-NMR spectral data. Some of these compounds showed leishmanicidal activity.
>
> PMID: 19252314 [PubMed - indexed for MEDLINE]   Free full text

Vascular

Blimey we are rocking up the long words today.

Artherogenisis is seen as a main cause of not only heart disease but any illness which includes the vascular system. It is thought that it causes the cholesterol plaque build up that lines the walls of the blood vessels, narrowing them and impeding health. In 2005, it was validated that *HPLC purified polyphenolic fraction IV of Tulsi* may have profound antiarthrogenic effects. (In this case it is kind of essential oil that has been messed about with a bit. Tulsi, nevertheless)

Again now cutting edge research, only six days old at the time of writing, is the validation by The University of Florida that Holy Basil will slow the hardening of arteries, or *atherosclerosis* . It has been identified that the process responsible for this aspect of vascular decline is an oxidant enzyme called *myeloperoxidase*. Again the golden boy was identified at euganol, but here it was found that he could work alone or in the full tulsi extract.

I like seeing the difference in the cultures here. In the Indian papers, they are happy to commit to strong conclusions of how tulsi helps this that and the other. In the land of litigation, Orlando researchers know to be a little more cautious…

"Based on these results, we conclude that basil extract could act as an inhibitor of MPO and may serve as a nonpharmacological therapeutic agent for atherosclerosis."

Could.

Remember that people, please.

It *could*.

We know it will execute the physiological processes required, but will that be enough to actually treat the problem at the global levels it would need to become a drug for instance…? We'll have to see. Regardless of that, what we can say is it is a herb that we now know protects the arteries.

> Abstract ▾
>
> J Med Food. 2015 Mar 12. [Epub ahead of print]
>
> **Therapeutic Potential of Ocimum tenuiflorum as MPO Inhibitor with Implications for Atherosclerosis Prevention.**
>
> Narasimhulu CA, Vardhan S.
>
> Author information
>
> Abstract
> Current experimental studies show that Ocimum tenuiflorum (commonly known as basil or Tulsi) possesses many health benefits. Ocimum is suggested to be antioxidative and anti-inflammatory. Eugenol, an orthomethoxyphenol, and ursolic acid have been identified as important components of basil. Myeloperoxidase (MPO), an oxidative enzyme, has been implicated in the pathogenesis of atherosclerosis. MPO-dependent oxidation of lipoproteins has been implicated in foam cell formation, dysfunctional HDL, and abnormalities in reverse cholesterol transport. Whole leaf extract of O. tenuiflorum and its major components, eugenol and ursolic acid, inhibit the oxidation of lipoproteins by myeloperoxidase/copper as measured by conjugated diene formation as well as by the thiobarbituric acid reactive substance (TBARS) assay. Whole basil leaf extract is able to attenuate the lipopolysaccharide-induced inflammation in RAW 264.7 cells compared with its components. In addition, whole basil leaf extract and eugenol inhibited MPO enzyme activity against synthetic substrates. Based on these results, we conclude that basil extract could act as an inhibitor of MPO and may serve as a nonpharmacological therapeutic agent for atherosclerosis.
>
> KEYWORDS: eugenol; inflammation; lipopolysaccharide; lipoproteins; oxidation; ursolic acid
>
> PMID: 25764050 [PubMed - as supplied by publisher]

Cholesterol

My anatomy and physiology is good enough for me to know I have put this in the wrong section and that it should be in the liver section really, because that's where cholesterol is formed but...

A very old trial from 1994 showed that rabbits who had feasted on Tulsi leaves for four weeks had reduced triglycerides, lipids and cholesterol in their blood.

> Abstract ▾
>
> Indian J Physiol Pharmacol. 1994 Oct;38(4):311-2.
>
> **Changes in the blood lipid profile after administration of Ocimum sanctum (Tulsi) leaves in the normal albino rabbits.**
>
> Sarkar A[1], Lavania SC, Pandey DN, Pant MC.
>
> Author information
>
> Abstract
> Administration of fresh leaves of Ocimum sanctum (Tulsi) mixed as 1 g and 2 g in 100 gms of diet given for four weeks, brought about significant changes in the lipid profile of normal albino rabbits. This resulted in significant lowering in serum total cholesterol, triglyceride, phospholipid and LDL-cholesterol levels and significant increase in the HDL-cholesterol and total faecal sterol contents.
>
> PMID: 7883302 [PubMed - indexed for MEDLINE]

Cancer

It is bizarre to think that this report was only posted seven days ago, as I write this. It really does show how fast this research is coming through now and, of course, that is not only down to the change in the way medicine views essential oils, but also progression in technology and the internet age. Communication and knowledge sharing is lightening fast, and so it should be, because how life changing will it eventually be when they are able to find a way to make a drug to treat prostate cancer from this plant. Researchers at Rumbaugh Goodwin Institute for Cancer Research from Fort Lauderdale in Florida have established that ethanoic acid extracted from Sacred Basil is able to fragment the DNA of cancerous prostate cells and to bring about cell death.

Abstract

J Med Food. 2015 Feb 18. [Epub ahead of print]

Apoptosis Induction by Ocimum sanctum Extract in LNCaP Prostate Cancer Cells.

Dhandayuthapani S[1], Azad H, Rathinavelu A.

Author information

Abstract

Tulsi (Ocimum sanctum Linn), commonly known as "holy basil," has been used for the treatment of a wide range of ailments in many parts of the world. This study focuses on apoptosis-inducing ability of tulsi extract on prostate cancer cells. For this purpose LNCaP prostate cancer cells were treated with different concentrations of 70% ethanolic extract of tulsi (EET) and then the cytotoxicity was determined after 24 and 48 h. After treatment with EET externalization of phosphatidyl serine (PS) from the inner membrane to outer leaflet of the plasma membrane was clearly evidenced by the results obtained from both flow cytometry analysis with Annexin V-FITC and pSIVA-IANBD binding fluorescence microscopy assay. Depolarization of the mitochondrial membrane potential was also evidenced by the presence of 5,5',6,6'-tetrachloro-1,1',3,3'-tetraethyl benzimedazolyl carbocyanine iodide (JC-1) monomeric form in the EET-treated cells that emitted the green fluorescence when compared with the control cells that emitted the red fluorescence due to aggregation of JC-1. Furthermore, the level of poly (ADP-ribose) polymerase (PARP) cleavage and Bcl-2 were determined using western blot analysis. When compared to the control cells the level of cleaved PARP was found to be higher with a concomitant decrease in the Bcl-2 level after 24 h of treatment of cells with EET. In addition, treatment with EET significantly elevated the activities of caspase-9 and caspase-3 in LNCaP cells compared with the control. Also, after 48 h of treatment all doses used in this study showed clear fragments of DNA, which is one of the hallmarks of apoptosis. Taken together, our findings suggest that, EET can effectively induce apoptosis in LNCaP cells via activation of caspase-9 and caspase-3 that can eventually lead to DNA fragmentation and cell death.

KEYWORDS: Bcl-2; DNA fragmentation; LNCaP-prostate cancer; PARP-cleavage; apoptosis; caspases; mitochondrial membrane potential; pSIVA-IANBD; tulsi

PMID: 25692494 [PubMed - as supplied by publisher]

This augments the research established in 2011 that found then another active ingredient, the flavinoid *vicenin-2* helps to bring about cell death of the same prostate cancer cells.

> **Abstract**
>
> Biochem Pharmacol. 2011 Nov 1;82(9):1100-9. doi: 10.1016/j.bcp.2011.07.078. Epub 2011 Jul 23.
>
> **Anti-cancer effects of novel flavonoid vicenin-2 as a single agent and in synergistic combination with docetaxel in prostate cancer.**
>
> Nagaprashantha LD[1], Vatsyayan R, Singhal J, Fast S, Roby R, Awasthi S, Singhal SS.
>
> Author information
>
> [1] Department of Diabetes and Metabolic Diseases Research, Beckman Research Institute, City of Hope, National Medical Center, Duarte, CA 91010, USA.
>
> **Abstract**
>
> The present study was conducted to determine the efficacy of novel flavonoid vicenin-2 (VCN-2), an active constituent of the medicinal herb Ocimum Sanctum Linn or Tulsi, as a single agent and in combination with docetaxel (DTL) in carcinoma of prostate (CaP). VCN-2 effectively induced anti-proliferative, anti-angiogenic and pro-apoptotic effect in CaP cells (PC-3, DU-145 and LNCaP) irrespective of their androgen responsiveness or p53 status. VCN-2 inhibited EGFR/Akt/mTOR/p70S6K pathway along with decreasing c-Myc, cyclin D1, cyclin B1, CDK4, PCNA and hTERT in vitro. VCN-2 reached a level of 2.6±0.3μmol/l in serum after oral administration in mice which reflected that VCN-2 is orally absorbed. The i.v. administration of docetaxel (DTL), current drug of choice in androgen-independent CaP, is associated with dose-limiting toxicities like febrile neutropenia which has lead to characterization of alternate routes of administration and potential combinatorial regimens. In this regard, VCN-2 in combination with DTL synergistically inhibited the growth of prostate tumors in vivo with a greater decrease in the levels of AR, pIGF1R, pAkt, PCNA, cyclin D1, Ki67, CD31, and increase in E-cadherin. VCN-2 has been investigated for radioprotection and anti-inflammatory properties. This is the first study on the anti-cancer effects of VCN-2. In conclusion, our investigations collectively provide strong evidence that VCN-2 is effective against CaP progression along with indicating that VCN-2 and DTL co-administration is more effective than either of the single agents in androgen-independent prostate cancer.
>
> Copyright © 2011 Elsevier Inc. All rights reserved.
>
> PMID: 21803027 [PubMed - indexed for MEDLINE] PMCID: PMC3252753 Free PMC Article

Cancer Cells

> Abstract
>
> Cancer Biol Ther. 2013 May;14(5):417-27. doi: 10.4161/cbt.23762. Epub 2013 Feb 4
>
> **Ocimum gratissimum retards breast cancer growth and progression and is a natural inhibitor of matrix metalloproteases.**
>
> Nangia-Makker P[1], Raz T, Tait L, Shekhar MP, Li H, Balan V, Makker H, Fridman R, Maddipati K, Raz A.
>
> Author information
>
> Abstract
>
> Ocimum genus (a.k.a holy basil or tulsi) is a dietary herb used for its multiple beneficial pharmacologic properties including anti-cancer activity. Here we show that crude extract of Ocimum gratissimum (OG) and its hydrophobic and hydrophilic fractions (HB and HL) differentially inhibit breast cancer cell chemotaxis and chemoinvasion in vitro and retard tumor growth and temporal progression of MCF10ADCIS.com xenografts, a model of human breast comedo-ductal carcinoma in situ (comedo-DCIS). OG-induced inhibition of tumor growth was associated with decreases in basement membrane disintegration, angiogenesis and MMP-2 and MMP-9 activities as confirmed by in situ gelatin zymography and cleavage of galectin-3. There was also decrease in MMP-2 and MMP-9 activities in the conditioned media of OG-treated MCF10AT1 and MCF10AT1-EIII8 premalignant human breast cancer cells as compared with control. The MMP-2 and MMP-9 inhibitory activities of OG were verified in vitro using gelatin, a synthetic fluorogenic peptide and recombinant galectin-3 as MMP substrates. Mice fed on OG-supplemented drinking water showed no adverse effects compared with control. These data suggest that OG is non-toxic and that the anti-cancer therapeutic activity of OG may in part be contributed by its MMP inhibitory activity.
>
> **KEYWORDS:** Breast Cancer; MMP; Ocimum gratissimum; Tumor progression
>
> PMID: 23380593 [PubMed - indexed for MEDLINE] PMCID: PMC3672186 Free PMC Article

This one is incredibly confusing, so please try and stick with me. The first thing to point out is this is a different strain of Holy Basil. It is not *sanctum* or *tenuiflorum* but this time...gratissimum (Remember the Forest Tulsi?)

Again this is extracts of dried leaves extracted using methanol, but this time fractionalised again using two methods, hydrophobic and hydrophilic extraction. (Very simplistically explained, two reagents are added and then it is put into a centrifuge and they separate differently, one towards the water molecules and one away from....).

The extracts worked differently, one halting the cells' ability to cleave to the mast cell and the other preventing chemotaxis, which is the way the cancer cells travel and mutate. Working together it confirmed that extracts from tulsi are able to halt tumour growth.

So, a team in Karantaka wanted to answer the same question that I have been asking all the way along. What are the active ingredients that are doing this work? Euganol we know, but also they isolated that rosmarinic acid (which makes me think I need to be looking at rosemary research soon) apinegin (which is usually connected to treating anxiety, because it is one of the sedative components in camomile for example) and also carnosic acid. Carnosic acid again is found in the greatest quantities in rosemary and also sage. Other active constituents are listed below

```
Abstract ▼                                                                         Send to: ▼

Nutr Cancer. 2013;65 Suppl 1:26-35. doi: 10.1080/01635581.2013.785010.
Ocimum sanctum L (Holy Basil or Tulsi) and its phytochemicals in the prevention and treatment of cancer.
Baliga MS, Jimmy R, Thilakchand KR, Sunitha V, Bhat NR, Saldanha E, Rao S, Rao P, Arora R, Palatty PL.
⊞ Author information

Abstract
Ocimum sanctum L. or Ocimum tenuiflorum L, commonly known as the Holy Basil in English or Tulsi in the various Indian languages, is a important medicinal plant in the various traditional and folk systems of medicine in Southeast Asia. Scientific studies have shown it to possess antiinflammatory, analgesic, antipyretic, antidiabetic, hepatoprotective, hypolipidemic, antistress, and immunomodulatory activities. Preclinical studies have also shown that Tulsi and some of its phytochemicals eugenol, rosmarinic acid, apigenin, myretenal, luteolin, β-sitosterol, and carnosic acid prevented chemical-induced skin, liver, oral, and lung cancers and to mediate these effects by increasing the antioxidant activity, altering the gene expressions, inducing apoptosis, and inhibiting angiogenesis and metastasis. The aqueous extract of Tulsi and its flavanoids, orintin, and vicenin are shown to protect mice against γ-radiation-induced sickness and mortality and to selectively protect the normal tissues against the tumoricidal effects of radiation. The other important phytochemicals like eugenol, rosmarinic acid, apigenin, and carnosic acid are also shown to prevent radiation-induced DNA damage. This review summarizes the results related to the chemopreventive and radioprotective properties of Tulsi and also emphasizes aspects that warrant future research to establish its activity and utility in cancer prevention and treatment.

PMID: 23082780 [PubMed - indexed for MEDLINE]
```

The report goes on to explain that the protection against skin, liver, oral and lung cancers arises because of the anti-oxidant properties of the herb and the way it can combat the effects of radiation. Most precisely we know that carnosic acid has the capability to protect against radiation in its own right.

Anti Genotoxic

It's time for us to go all Erin Brockovich now. Can you remember when Julia Roberts told the story of Hinkley and its dreadful health demise from hexavalent chromium in 1993?

Researchers at National Environmental Engineering Research Institute in Nagpur wanted to assess how tulsi might affect the way hexavalent chromium (and another chemical, mytomycin C) broke human DNA strands, leading to the cell changes (genotoxicity) that would eventually lead to cancer.

Tulsi essential oil was able to reduce the effects of mitomycin C by 69% and hexovalent chromium by 71%. Chromosomes forming in a petri dish were protected and micronuclei formed more healthily. Here, the anti-oxidant properties were attributed to eugenol, luteolin and apigenin.

Those poor people in Hinkley. How sad that this information was uncovered less than two decades later. That makes me both sad and hopeful at the same time.

> **Biomed Environ Sci.** 2007 Jun;20(3):226-34
>
> ### Modulatory effect of distillate of Ocimum sanctum leaf extract (Tulsi) on human lymphocytes against genotoxicants.
>
> Dutta D[1], Devi SS, Krishnamurthi K, Kumar K, Vyas P, Muthal PL, Naoghare P, Chakrabarti T.
>
> Author information
>
> [1]Environmental Biotechnology Division, National Environmental Engineering Research Institute (NEERI), Nehru Marg, Nagpur - 440020, India. dipanwita.dd@gmail.com
>
> #### Abstract
>
> **OBJECTIVE:** To study the modulatory effect of distillate of Ocimum sanctum (traditionally known as Tulsi) leaf extract (DTLE) on genotoxicants.
>
> **METHODS:** In the present investigation, we studied the antigenotoxic and anticlastogenic effect of distillate of Tulsi leaf extract on (i) human polymorphonuclear leukocytes by evaluating the DNA strand break without metabolic activation against mitomycin C (MMC) and hexavalent chromium (Cr+6) and (ii) human peripheral lymphocytes (in vitro) with or without metabolic activation against mitomycin C (MMC), hexavalent chromium (Cr+6) and B[a]P by evaluating chromosomal aberration (CA) and micronucleus assay (MN). Three different doses of DTLE, 50 microL/mL, 100 microL/mL, and 200 microL/mL were selected on the basis of cytotoxicity assay and used for studying DNA strand break, chromosomal aberration and micronucleus emergence. The following positive controls were used for inducing genotoxicity and clastogenicity: MMC (0.29 micromol/L) for DNA strand break, chromosomal aberration and 0.51 micromol/L for micronucleus assay; Potassium dichromate (Cr+6) 600 micromol/L for DNA strand break and 5 micromol/L for chromosomal aberration and micronucleus assay; Benzo[a]pyrene (30 micromol/L) for chromosomal aberration and 40 micromol/L for micronucleus assay. The active ingredients present in the distillate of Tulsi leaf extract were identified by HPLC and LC-MS.
>
> **RESULTS:** Mitomycin C (MMC) and hexavalent chromium (Cr+6) induced statistically significant DNA strand break of respectively 69% and 71% (P<0.001) as revealed by fluorometric analysis of DNA unwinding. Furthermore, the damage could be protected with DTLE (50 microL/mL, 100 microL/mL, and 200 microL/mL) on simultaneous treatment. Chromosomal aberration and micronucleus formation induced by MMC, Cr+6 and B[a]P were significantly protected (P<0.001) by DTLE with and without metabolic activation.
>
> **CONCLUSION:** Distillate of Tulsi leaf extract possesses antioxidants contributed mainly by eugenol, luteolin and apigenin as identified by LC-MS. These active ingredients may have the protective effect against genotoxicants.
>
> PMID: 17672214 [PubMed - indexed for MEDLINE]

Now, for the bad news...

Well it depends on the size on your family I suppose. It might be good news. It is certainly good news for farmers who are losing all their lettuces to pesky rabbits. Tulsi reduces sperm count, sperm motility, and testes size.

This finding backed up suspicions derived from a 1992 study of male rats whose sexual behaviour *decreased* dramatically according to how much tulsi they consumed.

An easy crop to plant as a barrier to the fields and hmmm...as good as a vasectomy, I wonder....? (In these days of litigation I feel I must add that **Holy Basil should not be considered to be contraceptive and will not protect against**

sexually transmitted diseases or pregnancy...please use a condom).

Peter rabbit, however...

(Sorry darling, I have a headache tonight. You know what, how about I brew us both a nice cup of Holy Basil tea and I'll see how I feel later?)

Fish

Now, feel free to skip this last report because it is aquarium talk, but as many of you know we are fish mad in our house and I am fascinated to find how much essential oil data there is out there for tank heads. You might not use this, but possibly I will so...

Aeromonas hydrophilia gives fish dermatitis blisters under the skin and eventually (in about 2-3 weeks) kills them when it affects their haemoglobin levels and blood count. Again here we have ethanoic extractions and the fish were treated with a 1:1:1 ratio of turmeric, neem and tulsi. They were treated with a 1% dilution with a net into a hospital tank for 5 minutes on days 1, 3, 9 & 15. For clarification, this is a triherbal solution not any one herb. Restorative affects achieved!!!

> Abstract ▾   Send to: ▾
>
> J Aquat Anim Health. 2008 Sep;20(3):165-76. doi: 10.1577/H05-035.1
>
> **In vitro and in vivo studies of the use of some medicinal herbals against the pathogen Aeromonas hydrophila in goldfish.**
>
> Harikrishnan R[1], Balasundaram C.
>
> ⊕ Author information
>
> Abstract
>
> Aeromonas hydrophila is a ubiquitous and opportunistic bacterial pathogen that produces ulcerative dermatitis under stress conditions and inflicts severe losses on global fisheries and fish culture. This study evaluates the antimicrobial potency of aqueous and ethanolic decoction (individual extract) and concoction (mixed extract) of three common medicinal herbs, turmeric Curcuma longa, Tulsi plant Ocimum sanctum, and neem Azadirachta indica, against the in vitro growth of A. hydrophila. Among the decoctions, A. indica exhibited the most potent antibacterial property ($P < 0.05$) against A. hydrophila. Among the concoctions, both the aqueous and ethanolic triherbal extracts mixed in the ratio of 1:1:1 had higher antibacterial activity ($P < 0.05$) than the other concoctions and decoctions. Goldfish Carassius auratus (10 +/- 2 g) were challenged with A. hydrophila intramuscularly in the caudal region with two separate doses (days 1 and 3) of 50 microL/fish ($1.8 \times 10(3)$ colony-forming units per milliliter). On days 9 (early) and 15 (late) of infection, fish were held in a net and dip treated for 5 min daily in a 1-L solution of 1% aqueous triherbal concoction. Red blood cell (RBC) count, hemoglobin, and hematocrit levels of the infected group were significantly higher ($P < 0.05$) than those of the control group. In the early treated group, all of the affected profile values returned to near normal, while the late-treated group registered a partial recovery, such as improved RBC count. The derived hematological values, such as mean corpuscular volume, mean corpuscular hemoglobin, and mean corpuscular hemoglobin concentration, of the early and late-treated groups also significantly declined ($P < 0.05$) but were restored to near normal ($P > 0.05$) only in the early treated group. The results suggest that dip treatment of A. hydrophila-infected goldfish in an aqueous triherbal concoction had a synergistic restorative effect on the hematological variables.
>
> PMID: 18942593 [PubMed - indexed for MEDLINE]

(RIP beautiful white widow tetra. I wish I had known this before.)

Spiritual Aspects of Holy Basil

I am finding it very difficult to articulate the spiritual aspects of this oil because for the most part they are *too* big, too profound and, well, too holy really. It almost feels inadequate to try to put them into adjectives.

Whereas with other plants you can see a spiritual element alongside and interwoven in the physical healing, the medicine of *this* plant is goddess-like in *all* of its abilities. It seems to have magical potential to wash away psychic muck in ways I have never seen in any other oil.

An example here from my own life may probably help.

I have been writing *this* book amidst what I have described to my friends as "looking into the fires of hell". Someone I love very much has developed a hideously contorting and terrifying illness. It has flared from nowhere and is shocking to see but is also very shocking in its intensity.

To carry on working I have struggled to find a way to separate great angst from day to day life, and try to keep some semblance of sanity not only in my writing but in the family home.

Just fifteen days after first opening the hellish portal I was shocked to find myself back on the train to the hospital almost willingly facing the nightmare again.

As I looked out of the window at the sheet of rain coming down from a black cloud in the distance, I reflected on the *truly* awesome power of essential oils. Less than three weeks after being sure I could never face it again, the fear was gone. The terror was completely dissipated and a revitalised sense of purpose had taken its place. The compassion I feared might be smashed to smithereens was I found, entirely intact.

Followers of my blog will know how shocked I was at the potency of the tranquilising effects of spikenard and vetiver after the event, but strangest of all the actions does seem to have been Holy Basil.

I re-became me.

I can't think of a better way to describe it. Often an experience that scares you so much would leave a scar, more fear, anxiety, aggression, defensiveness...you might expect any of those to emerge. But they haven't. I feel exactly as if someone hit the reset button. My brain has discovered a great deal of things, and the knowledge is pure. It has grown from experience but is untarnished by the negative emotions that, to be honest, it really *should* have taken on.

The memory is still there. I can replay every moment, but where normally the amygdala would capture and replay it like a stuck record because of the dopamine cocktail it created, instead it is stored and happily filed away. It's almost like it happened to someone else, or it has been played out in a film (Shirley McLaine plays me, obviously!)

It seemed to me that the rain that I could see pouring in the distance was where I was about to go, the dark place. But just as the train was passing through it into the spring sunshine, I felt that essential oils guaranteed that I could go in, face the fear and come out again untouched.

Fire-walking, if you like.

Today, I find that I was right. I am tired and frazzled and do have the aura of a cartoon cat with its tail in the socket…but I am here, writing, and I am ok. I can feel yesterday dissipating even as I write.

During the train ride I read a few chapters of Michael S Gazzaniga's *Nature's Mind- The Biological Roots of Thinking, Emotions, Sexuality, Language and Intelligence* and was struck by a truth written as the very last sentence of the preface.

"They [societies] tend to succeed when they allow each individual to discover what millions of years' evolution has already bestowed on mind and body".

Just as biologists now agree that immunity does not develop, but rather we all carry every antibody in our system (and always have), the body simply has to select the correct one for the job, neurobiologists suspect that the same might be true of the brain. That is we do not ever learn anything new, more that everything we ever learn is merely discovering something your brain already had the capacity to do.

I began to wonder if rather than evolving as medicines the knowledge in plants is primordial and it is only now that *we* have found ways to select the triggers that can help our bodies to heal.

Holy Basil completely stripped back the vicious shock response that my body had engineered, it removed the chemical fear reply and calmed the hormones connected with it. When the layer of the emotional onion was peeled away the lower layers were found to be only very slightly affected by the surface trauma.

Added to that a strange series of events that led me to even research the oil makes me stop and consider who or what even put it in my hands at all.

In February I was asked by the Hungarian magazine Aromatika.hu to write a piece on Basil, which would never have occurred to me at all. It seemed like a really uninspired choice to me, and yet when I started to consider the oil, it was brought to life. The investigations led me to Holy Basil, which I knew was an oil, but I had never used so I decided to study it. When I collect data on any oil, my process is always the same, to use it and witness how it affects not only me but those around me too. I ordered the oil and it was delivered through my letter box on the Thursday and on Saturday all hell broke loose...

So...

How come the very oil I needed was suddenly in my box?

Hmmm, that dear reader might be completely co-incidence or Divine Intervention?

We'll never know.

Either way, I am grateful of it.

There is a very astute but gentle teaching quality to Holy Basil in that it focuses the mind. This especially true of using it in meditation, in yoga or in Quigong. In everyday life though, you can concentrate ion work better and avoid distractions that might get in the way. It quietens the mind, and the biproduct of this is you become far more aware of inspiration and your inner voice.

Emotional aspects of Basil

As ever we have this strange cross over between the three bodies. Holy Basil seems to be able to dissipate the mental fog that can be connected with Attention Deficit Disorder. Do we say this is physical, mental or emotional...I am not sure really. All of the above, I suppose.

Certainly it opens the heart to be more receptive to God.

It engenders faith, clarity and compassion. It increases goodness in a soul and shines a light of virtue and of joy.

Outside of the religious sense and moving more towards the spiritual, holding the mirror up to soul it is extremely helpful in gaining clarity about your true nature or purpose in this life.

Its sattvic nature purifies the body, mind and spirit, and brings harmony between the three. (Perhaps this is obvious, perhaps not, once the three are in balance a far better sense of wellness is achieved. It is an imbalance of these that we refer to as dis-ease.

I have deliberately not used the most dramatic of her names until now. Tulsi is the **Destroyer of Demons** and as such she is extraordinary in her capability with trauma. Somehow she seems to be able to collect together parts of the soul that have fragmented because of trauma. She seems to be able to reintegrate memories and experiences to be able to take a person to a new place of wholeness. She finds a way to locate lost souls and to bring them home. Remember what I had said about learning through experience but not having to carry the trauma with me? This is indeed Sacred Basil's energy.

It makes me laugh when I meditate with Tulsi because I keep hearing a set of lyrics from Prince "Coming in through the outdoor…" (*Raspberry Beret*). I didn't take much notice the first time it came through because I thought it was my mind wandering off unaccompanied again, but then I realised what it was. The soul has two pathways with Ocimum sanctum. Usually we see healing of this most divine nature only coming in through the crown chakra, and being pulled down through the root, but here, it also comes in through the root and it jam packs all the etheric bodies into a more stable arrangement...no more terrified cat...the energies are all concertina'd in.

Kapha energy can be stubborn, slow and we could say self sabotaging really. You can take this expressive element a bit further too, because many people turn to self sabotaging behaviour rather than dealing with negative emotions. Holy basil invigorates kapha to put a stop to comfort eating, for example. Kapha will often go out of kilter when the weather has been cold for a long time (bowl of stew anyone?) and so its warm, comforting hug puts paid to that behaviour.

In the same way, it pulls the emotional crutch from under you and boots you off the couch, switches off day time TV and demands you go and do something far healthier instead.

Chakras

There is a fine line between thoroughness and repetition in these books and I think the chakra section is possibly one of the areas most under threat of this. This medicine is covered at length in The Essential Oils of The Mind Body Spirit, and to avoid boring regular readers by coving old ground again, might I suggest you visit that book if this area is unfamiliar to you. Having said that, please do not take that as an inference that I feel this is not an important area of healing. Quite the reverse in fact, to my mind the subtle energies are the most advanced healing mechanism you can employ.

According to the Ayuvedic master Vasant Lad, Holy Basil is balancing and toning to the *all* the chakras. On the surface I expected it to open the crown but actually it almost feels like energy is being pulled like parachute strings in a cat's cradle. All of them are tugged and the energy seems to end up, right out in front of you just between the heart and the throat chakras.

When you consider the clinical data, you can see just how effectively this works. It touches pretty much every system of the body.

In particular you might notice:

How it affects metabolism through chakra 3. Here we see self worth issues too.

How it opens the heart chakra 4 to make it more receptive to love and compassion, both receiving and giving. It also protects on the physical level through the circulatory system and the heart.

Very importantly it has physical and emotional ties to chakra 5. There is a particular affinity with the mouth, but also through communication, not just with others but with one's own inner self.

As the energy rises through the chakras and the compassion and goodness flows through the heart, then inner truth radiates through the throat chakra and soon inspiration and spiritual cleansing can be seen through the third eye, or brow chakra. Most importantly there is a far better perception of knowing one's own mind here.

Eventually chakra 7 is vitalised allowing clear communication with one's god.

Unlike Monarda oil though, which has you "floating off on butterfly wings" Tulsi is extremely grounded and I suppose we might say this is where chakras 1 & 2 come in. After all the plant is the Earthly incarnation of a goddess. In the very truest sense of the word, it is grounded.

Ruling Planet
Being a plant of such abundance and blessing Holy Basil falls under the rulership of Jupiter. Certainly this is an astrological influence but it represents far more than simple metaphysical astrology. Nicolas Culpepper was reputed to have said that the

only physicians he would trust were those who had an understanding of the planets, but these attributions have a deeper more profound connection.

The eminent psychologist Carl Jung spoke of how every one of us has archetypes running right through the core of our psyches. These are deeply ingrained patterns of symbols that hold the same sets of values to each of us regardless of religion or culture.

Everything about Jupiter energy feels wonderful. It is expansive, growing, blessing. He brings belief integrity and trust into our lives. He is elevating and uplifting. We can see expansion in three ways here, all of which are true. **Expansion of beliefs and a sense of the greater universe**, **expansion in the bulge of your wallet** and actual material wealth and **expansion of your girth**! Jupiter will always lead to a larger tummy if you are not careful.

His shadow side is greed, avarice and pride and think about how Holy Basil gives you that almighty kick up the behind and do something. Most certainly, Holy Basil does not like self sabotaging!!! It's worth thinking about what these indulgences can lead to physically, heart disease, cholesterol and stomach ulcers...all Holy Basil complaints!

It is strange too that one of the lessons of Jupiter is how we can happily go along the wrong path without introspection. We get the money and the riches and then suddenly wake up one morning and wonder "How on Earth did I get here?" The hollow ring of the factory bell in the job you hate is very much Jupiter medicine…and it tends not to be delivered very subtly either. Conversely, can you see how Holy Basil allows you dwell on the questions of "**Who am I?**" and "**What do I want?**" quietly and effectively? That very clear mirror reflects the desires of your spirit…not the say so of the pay check.

Most relevantly Jupiter allows us to make more mistakes than many of the other planets because he wants us to learn from them. It is only from experience that we can move forward…and that's quite a familiar lesson too, really, too isn't it?

When Jupiter energy is flowing it is optimistic and positive, but when the energy drops then you will see self righteousness and pompous attitudes.

Anyone got a bottle of Holy Basil to hand?

Jupiter is about power, authority and direction. If there are questions about "I don't know what I want…" or "I can't" (especially if it is coupled by actions which may seem to be bullying in order to compensate) then there are definitely Jupiter lessons happening and Holy Basil will help. "I can't" of course, is often as a result of a traumatic fall from grace or failure in the past, which is easily neutralised with ocimum sanctum.

Remember too that Jupiter is an expression of Zeus, the king of the gods. Again we have this sense of the elite about the plant!

Chapter 5 The Essential Oil

There seems to be three schools of thought as to where the magic comes from in terms of its chemistry. Without doubt its high levels of euganol are extremely important and are what sets Holy Basil apart from other members of the Ocimum family. Gas spectrometry readings show that for many sources it makes up over 50% of the oil with Caryophyllene offering up just under a third more of the constituency. These also mean that the oil may be irritant to many skins and so must only be used in very low dilutions; not more than 1%.

Rosmarinic acid seems to be reason for its antioxidant potency and linalool is responsible for its anti-fungal prowess.

Extraction
Steam distillation from leaves and seeds

Yield
Typical yield is about 8%

Safety Data
Ocimum Tenuiflorum L.

Ocimum Sanctum L.

Tisserand and Young 2013 suggest maximum dosage of 1% dilution for dermal usage although IFRA regulations say 0.5%. I would be inclined to agree that 1% is best here, certainly no more because of the high euganol content.

Forest Tulsi

Ocimum gratissimum L

Probable dermal irritant. According to Tisserand and Young 2013 do not use in dilutions of strong than 0.2%

*Both strains of Tulsi (tenuiflorum and grattissimum) should be **used with care** if the patient is also taking **anti-coagulant blood medication** (because of its tonic effects on the vascular system) or **diabetes medication.** Ask your physician for support and guidance with this.*

Do not use any essential oils from the Basil family in the first 16 weeks of pregnancy.

Distribution

Across the globe but naturally the biggest producer is India

Blending

Holy basil has a very strong scent. It is sharp, almost minty with a camphorous and herbaceous fragrance. At times it can be almost sweetly spicy with a balsamic undertone and it then dries down to be reminiscent of cloves (which I suspect is the euganol coming through).

It is a **Top-Middle** note and in yin neutral. (See The Professional Stress Solution.)

It blends well with florals, bergamot, clary sage, geranium, hyssop, lime, black pepper, opoponax, cedarwood, citronella, fennel, ginger, grapefruit, lavender, lemon, marjoram, neroli and verbena.

How to meditate with Tulsi

I don't feel it is my place to regale all the prayers to Lakshmi. It should be a Hindu that reveals those. There are some beautiful ones. I have included a link in the resources to that page with the ones I love though.

Using the oil as a means of accessing the inner space of your mind though, although still arcane, I feel more comfortable sharing.

As you know I am not one for sitting cross legged for many hours, but I must confess to finding it far easier when I used this oil. I recommend using a piece of music as a means to anchor your counting and then simply *be* with the music . use Yiruma's gorgeous "The River Flows through you". It is amazing how simply you can centre your awareness this way.

Counting in cycles of 8, breath in and then out and then in again; focus on your breathing and the ebb and flow of the music, nothing else.

I think it is important to say, don't worry if your mind wanders. Try (in fact, *don't* try, if that makes sense) to watch it from detachment as if it is happening to someone else. Simply observe how it trickles and meanders. It will start off thinking about what's for tea and whether you can get the washing dry but after a while the domestic clutter will pass and in the quietness of your mind you may find a voice speaks whom you haven't heard for a long time. Your inner voice, the true voice, the essence of you.

Listen.

Don't strain to hear. Just observe....and don't forget to smile. You want her to keep coming back don't you? After all how long has it been since you met this old friend.

I find that She returns even when I least expect her. Listen to the same music in the bath, perhaps. She'll come to her trigger. Ask her to come in your dreams. Pray for guidance on where your path should be.

Remember though, Lakshmi has four things in her hands. Whilst She brings Moksha and enlightenment, her gifts are also pure joy and love. She is exuberant and explosive. Yes there is contentment, but also there is celebration. Surely the greatest meditations come through song and dance?

Vibration

Colour

Yellow

Musical Note

A Major

Doing this part of the book is always my favourite bit because when I finally put the music on to check whether I have got the right resonance in my head, it feels like an explosion when the oil and musical notes come together. With this one ...fireworks went off! Not least because I realised those strange words "*She came in through the outdoor*" had been a clue all along.

Raspberry Beret is written in the key of A Major, the vibratory note of Holy Basil. It is a strange almost enigmatic key where every note sounds very strangely off, but still right, all the same.

The most elegant portrayal of this is in my favourite song from my teenage years Robert Palmer's *She Makes My Day*, Tracey Chapman's *Fast Car*, Snow Patrol's *Chasing Cars*, REO Speedwagon's *Can't Fight This Feeling Any More* are all written in the same key. Somehow, even in the calm and melancholy melodies joy shines through.

Classical pieces include Joseph Hayden's *Symphony Number 59 "Fire"* and my personal recommendation for meditation the stunningly beautiful *"River Flows in You"* played by Yiruma.

To capture that sheer joy of Indian celebration, how about Dancing Queen by ABBA, Beautiful Day by U2 or Shake your Groove Thing Peaches and Herb. Just because there is an essential oil diffusing, doesn't mean we have to be quiet and contemplate....release your soul and dance like no-one is watching!!!

Recipes

As ever, I am going to remind you that the very best therapy comes from your own intuition and insights into each individual patient; it almost never comes off a recipe sheet. That being said using only 1% dilution of Holy Basil means it is going to last you a *loooong* time!

1 x = 1 drop

Please refer to The Complete Guide to Clinical Aromatherapy and The Essential Oils of The physical Body for notes on blending and application. Please don't feel you have to restrict yourself to these blends. Get creative, get innovative and above all become a healer. Recipes will teach you none of that, your own intuition will!

So here's some I made earlier

Diffuser blends:

Someone undermines your mission and dream

1 x Holy Basil

1 x Monarda

1 x Vetiver

Finances are scaring the pants off you!

1x Holy Basil

1 x Geranium

1 x Neroli

Parents are poorly

1 x Holy Basil

1 x Angelica

1 Frankincense

Exams are looming on the horizon

1 x Holy Basil

1 x Rosewood/ Ho Wood (better sustainable resource)

1 x vetiver

Bath to stop you self sabotaging

1 x Holy Basil

1 x Frankincense

1 x cypress

Detox lotion to rid the body of food chemicals

100 ml (4 oz) lotion

1 x Holy Basil

1 Oregano

1 x Thyme

Use a small finger full daily and rub onto the inside of the wrist.

Lotion for Constipation

100 ml (4 oz) lotion

1 x Holy Basil

1 x Cardamom

2 x Ginger

Massage into the abdomen in a clockwise motion until well absorbed. Use as often as required. This should be about 10 treatments.

Catarrh Facial Massage Oil

25ml Sunflower oil

1 x Holy Basil

1 x Myrrh

1 x Frankincense

Massage around the sinuses and over the forehead. Use the facial massage treatment outlined in The Complete Guide to Clinical Aromatherapy and The Essential Oils of The Physical Body

Astringent Toner for Oily Skin

100 ml (4 fl oz) Orange Flower water

25 ml (1 fl oz) witch hazel

1 x Holy basil

1 x Linden Blossom Absolute

1 x Petitgrain

Use to cleanse the complexion morning and evening.

Lotion to Regulate Blood sugar

100 ml (4 oz) lotion

1 x holy Basil

1 x dill

1 x fennel

1 x rosemary

Use a finger full three times a day on the wrist. **Consult with your physician before using this blend. Do not use this unless you have the facility to check your blood sugars as it could fall dangerously low with your insulin too. Do NOT stop taking your insulin.**

Prayer of Gratitude

Within each and every Hindu house grows a Tulsi plant which it is required be watered and cleaned (only by women) every day. As they care for it, this prayer is offered.

Tulsi Devi Stuti

Thulasi shree sakhi shubhe, papa haarini punyade,
Namasthe Naradanuthe, Namo Narayana priye.

Oh, Holy Thulasi,
Bosom friend of Lakshmi,
Destroyer of sins,
Bestower of blessings,
Salutations to thee,
Who is praised by sage Narada,
And is the darling of Lord Narayana

Tulsi Gayatri Mantra

Om Tulsi devyai cha Vidhmahe
Vishnu priyayai cha Dheemahe
Thanno Brindah Prachodayath.

Om, Let me meditate on the Goddess of Ocimum, Oh, Goddess who is dear to Vishnu, give me higher intellect, And let Brindha illuminate my mind.

Authors comment.

Wow, what a plant!

I hope you have found some of what I have written useful and it has helped you to step outside of the more standard oils you see on sale.

It is nice to see a plant so deeply ensconced in religion that clearly it will always have a sustainable future and whether people realise how much of its healing they are absorbing or not, in this case really does not matter. It is an entire culture housed in a set of leaves and I think that is truly wonderful.

I want to offer a massive thanks to Chris Hackett, for whom I wrote this book. She is a newcomer to oils and answering all the questions and fantastic comments she places on social networks has become a full time job in itself! I love that she has become so engaged in aromatherapy and I hope some others of you will follow suit.

As ever thanks again to all of you who are buying my books and placing reviews on Amazon. Not only does it help to keep the pennies coming in but it helps me to understand what kind of books you want to read.

My next two books are Sweet Basil and Patchouli and I also have several orders for different pieces of work on Rose. It feels like spring maybe rather sweet this year. I hope yours will be too.

See you on the other side, and don't forget….
Review and Buy

Bye!
Liz

Resources

Bollywood's finest rendition of Tulsi Vivah celebratory dance. Notice the Holy Basil in the midst of the celebrations.
https://www.youtube.com/watch?v=5pfABe8A1Ik

An explosion of colour as a Hindu temple opens its doors to see a traditional celebration of *Tulsi vivah* from start to finish
https://www.youtube.com/watch?v=hPM22A6y00M

Beautiful page of sixteen stages of worship to Lakshmi with Holy Basil for Diwali
http://www.drikpanchang.com/festivals/lakshmipuja/info/lakshmi-puja-vidhi.html

Other books in The Secret Healer Series

The Essential Oils Profiles

<u>Vetiver</u>

<u>Monarda</u>

Coming soon....

Basil

Cedarwood

Sandalwood

Patchouli

To get the very best from your learning experience, why not treat yourself to one of the Secret Healer Training Manuals? To begin with, have you taken advantage of the free essential oil profiles available in...

<u>*Book 1 - The Complete Guide to*</u>

<u>*Clinical Aromatherapy & Essential Oils for the Physical Body*</u>

Essentially...essential oils for beginners, talented novices and intermediate aromatherapists

Let me ask you, why do you want a book on aromatherapy?

Do you want to learn how to care for your family naturally?

Perhaps you have a franchise selling essential oils and want to know more about what they can do?

Maybe you love the delicious scents and want understand how these beautiful things come to heal.

I wonder if you have started to learn and now want to discover how to build on your knowledge.

Whatever you are looking for this book has something for you.

- Details of how to treat over 60 conditions with essential oils
- Profiles of over 100 natural plant essences and their safety data
- Descriptions of 15 carrier oils and their applications not only for massage but also adding to creams and lotions.
- Comprehensive data of how the chemistry of an oil will affect its actions
- In depth insights into how professional aromatherapists blend…including their 13 favourite recipes from their practices.

Including….

- Sensuous aromatherapy blends by a qualified sex therapist
- Two blends for labour by the midwife running an aromatherapy program on an NHS maternity ward

- A blend for depression by a qualified mental health

PLUS....

10 bonus essential oil monographs and a complementary hypnotherapy relaxation download.

Discount vouchers of treatments courses and products by participating therapists.

AND.... for those of you who would like to contribute, there is a chance to make a donation to cancer research too.

This is my gift to you.

__Download for FREE - From 30.11.14__

Book 2 Essential Oils for Mind Body Spirit
The Holistic Medicine of Clinical Aromatherapy

Healing the skin, easing the tummy ache or getting someone to sleep is easy with essential oils. Anyone can do it. The joy of healing, though, comes from peeling back the layers of the disease, almost like a detective to find out exactly what caused it in the first place.

Consider this book to be lesson 2 in The Secret Healer Series.

You have mastered which oil to use for what and why...this book takes you step by step though the ancient healing mechanisms of the aura, the chakras and meridians but also explores how that ties in with the latest scientific discoveries into how the emotions affect our health. Using Candace Pert's remarkable "Molecules of Emotion" research, The Secret Healer shows you *where* to look for healing links and *why*.

- Uncover how a certain recurrent negative emotion can be the trigger to make you ill?
- Understand internal processes that mean that psychology, neurology and immunology are quintessentially, and inextricably linked.
- Learn how to use essential oils control your emotions and in turn bring about a far greater standard of wellness.
- Discover mindblowing research that shows the emotions we experience are actually the sensations of neuropeptides triggering our organs to do their jobs
- Reflect on the wonder of Chinese medicine and ancient healing being completely accurate in their healing mechanisms for thousands of years…now that science proves it to be so.

Essential Oils for The Mind Body Spirit couples ancient wisdom with cutting edge science. This is the knowledge the drug companies hope you never find out and our doctors pray we all will.

A short write up, for a book that will change your life. I promise you, when you read the latest findings of psychoneuroimmunology, you will never waste another day on being angry again.

Book 3 The Essential Oil Liver Cleanse
The Professional Aromatherapist's Liver Detox

We are warned of the threats of heart attacks, strokes and cancer, especially if we are overweight.

What is kept quieter is doctors have established a link between toxicity in the liver and metabolic syndrome, the condition that leads to many of these conditions. What's more non fatty liver disease is known to underlie many other conditions such as eczema, allergies and headaches.

The scandal is just how many of our livers are struggling under the strain of over processed foods, pharmaceutical debris and actually even our own bad tempers!

This book explains:

- The importance of the liver and its functions
- How it becomes dysfunctional and how to interpret warning signposts
- How to cleanse and nourish using not just essential oils, but also vitamins and minerals and diet.

- The strange correlation between how our emotions translate negativity into disease.
- How to implement other therapies such as chiropractic, acupressure and counselling and how to secure fantastic referrals.

This book is best used in tandem with The Professional Stress Solution to benefit from the complementary healing. Use Sales Strategies for Gentle Souls to create a marketing plan to use your new found knowledge to smash your competition out of the water!!!

Book 4 The Professional Stress Solution
Essential Oils and Holistic Health Stress Management Techniques for The Professional Aromatherapist

Stress is pandemic in our society.

Scientists agree it plays a quintessential role in how likely it is we will suffer from chronic and possibly fatal illnesses in the future. Risk factors of metabolic syndrome, diabetes, stroke and heart disease are increased through stress.

The daft thing is....aromatherapy can do amazing things to ease it, and potentially aromatherapists could take a massive workload away from the doctors' surgeries.

- Discover the hormonal changes and peptide triggers that change a person's health and mental state.
- Learn how it affects the liver, adrenals and pituitary gland.
- Uncover the strange phenomenon of Yin disease
- Build a better foundation of care, but also a knowledge base that means you can sell your treatments more effectively.
- Improve your healing skills set
- Supercharge your referrals potential from other complementary therapists and orthodox medicine alike.

Includes free bonus material of

- Chiropractic chart of misalignments and potential organic disturbance
- Chart of the meridians and suggested acupressure points to detox the organs more quickly
- Detailed information about how to improve the patients condition with vitamin and minerals therapy
- In depth dietary advice
- Free hypnotherapy relaxation download

Essential Oils are The Off Switch for stress. The *Professional Stress Solution* is the ON SWITCH for your aromatherapy business.

Book 5 The Aromatherapy Eczema Treatment

Healing Eczema, Itchy Skin Rashes and Atopic Dermatitis with Essential Oils and Holistic Medicine

Most people appreciate that the itching and redness of eczema can be used using essential oils, but what if I told you they were capable of so much more?

Imagine if, as a therapist, you were able to pinpoint the emotions that set off these flares? Can you visualise what it would mean to your patient if you were able to isolate the very protagonist causing the eczema breakout and alleviate their pain completely?

Well now you can.

This book teaches you:

- How to isolate the emotions causing the emotional cycle of pain
- The likely food triggers for your patient and the tools to identify the exact times they will detonate a reaction
- The familial traits and links that lead to atopic eczema
- How these links connect with the liver and in turn how to cleanse the liver toxicity
- Vitamins and minerals to cleanse and nourish the system

The book contains very real that will not only transform the way you treat clients, but will skyrocket your clinic's takings.

I recommend reading this book in tandem with *The Professional Stress Solution* and the *Essential Oil Liver Cleanse* to fully understand the cycles and processes of treatment. Add to it *Sales Strategies for Gentle Souls* and your business will stand on an entirely new footing.

Why not save yourself 1/3

And treat yourself to the set?

The full and comprehensive course into how to heal eczema

with aromatherapy and essential oils **$9.99 / £5.99**

The Aromatherapy Bronchitis Treatment

Support the Respiratory System with Essential Oils and Holistic Medicine for COPD, Emphysema, Acute and Chronic Bronchitis Symptoms

Breathing is the most natural thing in the world. It *should* be effortless, free and easy.
But if you are reading this...the chances are *your* breathing is not.

You are not alone. In fact COPD is **now the second biggest**

cause of death in the UK and the third in the United States. Respiratory disease is seriously bad news. Placing a massive burden on healthcare provision, **doctors place self care for respiratory disorders as one of their highest priorities**.

The question is…where on earth does one start?

Well, interestingly in these days of drug resistant bugs and infections, scientists are exploring respiratory medicine through a whole new realm…that of the plant kingdom. Over and over again they are finding that essential oils offer some of the best effects for bronchitis, emphysema and COPD.

Moreover, the scholars of psychoneuroimmunology have now concluded that the emotions (particularly from the past) play a vital role in the body's propensity to develop COPD, and that stress and hostility will assuredly make symptoms worse.

Together with detailed investigations into the essential oils to help maintain and support a healthy respiratory system, we look at how diet, emotional wellness and lifestyle changes can break the cycle of respiratory disease.

Some oils you may be able to guess; others are so unexpected they are like a bolt from the blue!

Discover:
- The essential oils found to be the most effective in **reducing inflammation, mucous and pain.**
- The hazardous oil able to positively affect Nitric Oxide, the gas considered vital to cardio vascular health and successful respiratory health.
- The foods suggested by doctors and nutritionists **to break the cycle of disease and support a healthier respiratory system**
- **Safe and clear instructions** on how to use which oil and when.
- Aromatherapy recipes to **clear infection, reduce pain, ease breathing and calm coughing.**

Sick of being sick...?
Relax...*breathe....we've got this covered.*
Improve your breathing, your sleep, even your emotional state and take the first steps on the road to getting your life back.
Clear, simple to follow advice and insights into your illness I'll bet you never even considered before!

Sales Strategies for Gentle Souls

Targeted Sales Training for Professional Aromatherapists

Wonderful things are happening in complementary therapy. Very gifted people are churning out fantastic research and results. The internet is full of what essential oils can do. But when a gentle soul emerges from their relaxing haze of their aromatherapy class room, how do they harness the buzz of energy around them for their craft?

From 1999-2008 I worked in one of the most aggressive commercial environments there is. My role as a recruitment consultant was 80% cold calling in an extremely saturated sales arena. Despite my own gentle soul, I found ways not only to compete, but to excel.

- Learn how to pinpoint the best customers for your practice
- Cost your treatments to ensure every treatment is profitable for both you and your customer
- Discover how to make every conversation into a potential sale lead without becoming a complete and utter pain in the a*s!
- Uncover the reasons why you are not closing sales so you never have to make the same mistakes again

- Create a growth environment where you plan success and always find yourself stepping into it

If you are working with essential oils, and you want to make a good living for it, then you need to learn to sell. What's more, if you are going to say "selling doesn't work on my customers"....then you have simply been taught to do it wrongly.

My dream is to see aromatherapy at the forefront of medicine. I need an army of gifted healers to achieve that. Consider yourself to be my newest recruit and I am going to drill you till you are the slickest, subtlest and most effective marketeer there is. You have the knowledge to make people better, now let me give you the business prowess to heal even more people than you have ever done before.

The Secret Healer has stress in her sights and she's about to make a killing. Listen carefully...she has much to tell you. £1.99 / $2.99

Buy now

www.thesecrethealer.co.uk

www.buildyourownreality.com

About the Author

Elizabeth Ashley qualified as an aromatherapist in 1993, and then passed her Advanced Aromatherapy Diploma in 1994. She has been practicing aromatherapy for almost 21 years.

In 1999, she fell into a whole new career in the aggressive commercial sector of recruitment consultancy. There she discovered her father's second hand car salesman genes had passed along and found she had quite a gift of the gab! More than that, she discovered she could sell…and then some.

In 2008, Elizabeth fell ill during pregnancy with a blood clot in her lungs. The pulmonary embolism prevented her from working and she started to write. Very quickly she gained her first contract as a ghost writer…a recipe book for cheese cakes!

In 2010 she was published professionally for her work on Galbanum oil in the Aromatherapy Thymes, journal of the International Federation of Aromatherapists, and on Tuberose oil by the New Zealand Register of Holistic Therapist.

In 2011 she was seconded on a consultative basis to Walsall Independent Treatment Centre, designed to be a rainbow bridge between traditional and complementary medicines. There she became aware of the rumblings of change in healthcare. Her book *Sales Strategies for Gentle Souls* explains the connotations of this.

Many of her books are aimed at helping qualified aromatherapists to expand their healing repertoire and build their businesses. She also writes for people who have an interest in essential oils and want to learn how to heal. Her in depth essential oil profiles chart the healing properties of plants from the most arcane depths of historic folklore up to the scientific lab trials of today.

In 2014 she ranks in the top 50 contract writers on the freelancer marketplace Elance.com. She is the ghost writer of seven number one Amazon best sellers in the natural healing category. She lives in Shropshire with her husband and youngest son, kept company by their cat, the budgie and many shoals of tropical fish! Her elder son and daughter attend University and make her prouder than anything ever could.

Elizabeth Ashley is possibly one of the most published aromatherapy writers you have never heard of! By 2015, all of that will have changed. Elizabeth Ashley is *The Secret Healer*.

Works Cited

(n.d.). Retrieved from http://www.grof-holotropic-breathwork.net/group/archetypalholotropicastrology/forum/topics/introduction-to-archetypal-1

Aggarwal K1, K. A. (2002, 06). *Knowledge, attitudes, beliefs and practices regarding measles in a rural area of Delhi.* Retrieved 03 18, 2015, from Pubmed: http://www.ncbi.nlm.nih.gov/pubmed/14768831

al., E. S. (2012, 02). *Diversified potentials of Ocimum sanctum Linn (Tulsi):An Exhaustive Survey.* Retrieved 03 02, 2015, from Scholars Research Library: http://scholarsresearchlibrary.com/jnppr-vol2-iss1/jnppr-2012-2-1-39-48.pdf

Babuji, P. (n.d.). *Prayer to Holy Basil.* Retrieved 03 30, 2015, from Namo nama Shri Guru padukabhyam: https://omshivam.wordpress.com/every-one-who-has-lost-hope-needs-vishwa-guru-ji%E2%80%99/prayer-to-tulsi-holy-basil/

Baliga MS1, J. R. (2013). *Ocimum sanctum L (Holy Basil or Tulsi) and its phytochemicals in the prevention and treatment of cancer.* Retrieved 03 17, 2015, from Pubmed: http://www.ncbi.nlm.nih.gov/pubmed/23682780

Benefits of Holy Basil . (2015). Retrieved 3 30, 2015, from Gentle Stress Relief.com: http://www.gentle-stress-relief.com/benefits-of-holy-basil.html

Biospiritual Healing Energy. (2012). *Holy Basil - The Mother Medicine of Nature.* Retrieved 03 30, 2015, from Biospiritual Healing Energy.com: http://www.biospiritual-energy-healing.com/holy-basil.html

Butler, R. (2009, 03 10). *Introduction to archetypal astrolog: Jupiter and Saturn.* Retrieved 03 29, 2015, from Holotropic breathwork Community: http://www.grof-holotropic-breathwork.net/group/archetypalholotropicastrology/forum/topics/introduction-to-archetypal-1

Chopra, D. (2015). *Tulsi Holy Basil.* Retrieved 03 30, 2015, from The Chopra Institute: http://www.chopra.com/tulsi-holy-basil

Coker, R. (2011, 12 16). *Roman Archetype Jupiter.* Retrieved 03 29, 2015, from Vitality Link: http://www.vitalitylink.com/article-palm-readers-palmistry-chirology-757-archetype-roman-god-jupiter-life-action

Dhandayuthapani S1, A. H. (2015, 02 18). *Apoptosis Induction by Ocimum sanctum Extract in LNCaP Prostate Cancer Cells.* Retrieved 02 25, 2015, from Pubmed: http://www.ncbi.nlm.nih.gov/pubmed/25692494

Floracopeia. (2015). *Tulsi- Holy Basil*. Retrieved 03 30, 2015, from Pubmed: http://www.floracopeia.com/Essential-Oils/essential-oils-sub/organic-tulsi-oil-holy-basil.html

Gianni, K. (2011, 03 20). *Holy Basil: My Number one Ace in the Hand, Herb For Adrenal Health*. Retrieved 03 30, 2015, from Renegade Health: http://renegadehealth.com/blog/2011/05/20/holy-basil-my-number-one-ace-in-the-hand-herb

Hakkim FL1, S. C. (2007, 10). *Chemical composition and antioxidant property of holy basil (Ocimum sanctum L.) leaves, stems, and inflorescence and their in vitro callus cultures*. Retrieved 03 30, 2015, from Pubmed: http://www.ncbi.nlm.nih.gov/pubmed/17924700

Halder N1, J. S. (2009, 12 23). *Ocimum sanctum extracts attenuate hydrogen peroxide induced cytotoxic ultrastructural changes in human lens epithelial cells*. Retrieved 03 17, 215, from Pubmed: http://www.ncbi.nlm.nih.gov/pubmed/19441070

Halim EM1, M. A. (2006, 09 21). *Effect ofOcimum sanctum (Tulsi) and vitamin E on biochemical parameters and retinopathy in streptozotocin induced diabetic rats*. Retrieved 03 17, 2015, from Halim EM1, Mukhopadhyay AK.: http://www.ncbi.nlm.nih.gov/pubmed/23105641

Harikrishnan R1, B. C. (2008, 09 20). *In vitro and in vivo studies of the use of some medicinal herbals against the pathogen Aeromonas hydrophila in goldfish*. Retrieved 03 17, 2015, from Pubmed: http://www.ncbi.nlm.nih.gov/pubmed/18942593

Helene, Z., & Kilham, C. (n.d.). *Holy Basil: Relieve Anxiety and Stress Naturally*. Retrieved 03 30, 2015, from Medicine Hunter: http://www.medicinehunter.com/holy-basil

Himalaya Wellness Since 1930. (2015). *Holy Basil*. Retrieved 03 30, 2014, from Himalaya Herbal Healthcare: http://himalayausa.com/products/pure-herbs/holy-basil

Holy Basil Tulsi Benefits. (n.d.). Retrieved 03 30, 2015, from Annies Remedy: http://www.anniesremedy.com/herb_detail464.php

India Essential Oils. (n.d.). *Natures Living Energy- Ocimum Sanctum*. Retrieved 03 30, 2015, from India Essential Oils: http://www.indiaessentialoils.com/holy-basil-oil.html

Iyenga, T. (2013). *Essence of Srivaishnavam Practices - Tulsi - Thulsi - Thulasi - तुलसी- துளஸி*. Retrieved 03 30, 2015, from TRS Iynega: https://www.trsiyengar.com/id34.shtml

Iyengar, T. (2015, 02 25). *Essence of Srivaishnavam Practices - Tulsi - Thulsi - Thulasi - तुलसी- துளஸி*. Retrieved 02 25,

2015, from Srivaishnavam Parambaryam, Traditions & The Culture that stands Class apart from others: https://www.trsiyengar.com/id34.shtml

J M A Hannan, L. M.-W. (2006, 04). *Ocimum sanctum leaf extracts stimulate insulin secretion from perfused pancreas, isolated islets and clonal pancreatic β-cells.* Retrieved 03 02, 2015, from Pubmed: http://joe.endocrinology-journals.org/content/189/1/127.long

Kantak NM1, G. M. (1992, 04). *Effect of short term administration of Tulsi (Ocimum sanctum Linn.) on reproductive behaviour of adult male rats.* Retrieved 03 18, 2015, from Pubmed: http://www.ncbi.nlm.nih.gov/pubmed/1506071

Khanna N1, B. J. (2003, 10). *Antinociceptive action of Ocimum sanctum (Tulsi) in mice: possible mechanisms involved.* Retrieved 03 18, 2015, from Pubmed: http://www.ncbi.nlm.nih.gov/pubmed/12963158

Lahon K1, D. S. (2011, 01). *Hepatoprotective activity of Ocimum sanctum alcoholic leaf extract against paracetamol-induced liver damage in Albino rats.* Retrieved 03 02, 2015, from Pubmed: http://www.ncbi.nlm.nih.gov/pubmed/21731390

lanetary Herbals. (n.d.). *Holy Basil*. Retrieved 03 30, 2015, from Planetary Herbals: http://www.planetaryherbals.com/products/GP2216/

Loon, G. V. (2009). *Chakara Samhita* . Retrieved 02 25, 2015, from Rencapp.com: http://www.rencapp.com/TamilCube_Charaka_Samhita.pdf

Mandal S1, D. D. (1993, 01). *Ocimum sanctum Linn--a study on gastric ulceration and gastric secretion in rats*. Retrieved 03 18, 2015, from Pubmed: http://www.ncbi.nlm.nih.gov/pubmed/8449557

Miracle Botanicals. (2014). *Tulsi- Holy Basil*. Retrieved 03 30, 2015, from Miracle Botanicals : https://miraclebotanicals.com/tulsi-holy-basil-essential-oil/

Mistry KS1, S. Z. (2014, 04 08). *The antimicrobial activity of Azadirachta indica, Mimusops elengi, Tinospora cardifolia, Ocimum sanctum and 2% chlorhexidine gluconate on common endodontic pathogens: An in vitro study*. Retrieved 02 25, 2015, from Pubmed: http://www.ncbi.nlm.nih.gov/pubmed/24966766

Mohammad S1, P. U. (2014, 01). *Herbal remedies for mandibular fracture healing*. Retrieved 02 25, 2015, from Pubmed: http://www.ncbi.nlm.nih.gov/pubmed/25298715

Montgomery, P. (2008). *Plant Spirit Healing*. Bear and Co.

Narasimhulu CA1, V. S. (2015, 03 12). *Therapeutic Potential of Ocimum tenuiflorum as MPO Inhibitor with Implications for Atherosclerosis Prevention*. Retrieved 03 18, 2015, from Pubmed: http://www.ncbi.nlm.nih.gov/pubmed/25764050

Natural Standard. (n.d.). *Holy Basil Ocimum sanctum.* Retrieved 03 30, 2015, from Whole Foods Market: http://www.livingnaturally.com/ns/DisplayMonograph.asp?storeID=E500FDE33212420DA51DB85BA6C3F8BA&DocID=bottomline-holybasil

Nature's Gift. (2014, 01 30). *GS Holy Basil Organic*. Retrieved 03 30, 2015, from Natures Gift: http://naturesgift.com/resources/gc/basil-holy-organic-india-2014-gc.pdf

New Zealand Hare Krishna Spiritual Resource Network. (2012, 11 12). *Tulasi Devi Links*. Retrieved 02 25, 2015, from New Zealand Hare Krishna Spiritual Resource Network: http://www.salagram.net/sstp-TulasiDevilinks.html

Oshadhi. (2015). *Holy Basil Organic Ocimum sanctum*. Retrieved 03 30, 2015, from Oshadhi: http://www.oshadhi.co.uk/holy-basil-organic-ocimum-sanctum/

Petruno, T. (n.d.). *Earth Medica: Healing Properties of Tulsi (Holy Basil)*. Retrieved 03 30, 2015, from Earth Energy Healings.com:

http://www.earthenergyhealings.com/blog/earth-medica-healing-properties-of-tulsi

Popham, S. (n.d.). *Pagyric Essences -Holy Basil.* Retrieved 03 30, 2015, from Organic Unity: http://www.organic-unity.com/products-page/spagyric-essences/ladys-mantle-spagyric-essence-duplicate/

Raja K1, P. A. (2014, 01). *In Silico Analysis to Compare the Effectiveness of Assorted Drugs Prescribed for Swine flu in Diverse Medicine Systems.* Retrieved 03 02, 2015, from Pubmed: http://www.ncbi.nlm.nih.gov/pmc/articles/PMC4007250/

Sage Meditation. (2015). *Tulsi Wood Prayer Beads* . Retrieved 03 30, 2015, from Sage Meditation: http://www.sagemeditation.com/tulsi-wood-meditation-mala-prayer-beads/

Saini A1, S. S. (2009, 04). *Induction of resistance to respiratory tract infection with Klebsiella pneumoniae in mice fed on a diet supplemented with tulsi (Ocimum sanctum) and clove (Syzgium aromaticum) oils.* Retrieved 03 17, 2015, from Pubmed: http://www.ncbi.nlm.nih.gov/pubmed/19597641

Sarkar A1, L. S. (1994, 10). *Changes in the blood lipid profile after administration of Ocimum sanctum (Tulsi) leaves in the normal albino rabbits.* Retrieved 03 18, 2015, from http://www.ncbi.nlm.nih.gov/pubmed/7883302

Suzuki A1, S. O. (2009, 03). *Leishmanicidal active constituents from Nepalese medicinal plant Tulsi (Ocimum sanctum L.).* Retrieved 03 17, 2015, from Pubmed: http://www.ncbi.nlm.nih.gov/pubmed/19252314

Disclaimer

by SEQ Legal

(1) Introduction

This disclaimer governs the use of this book. [By using this book, you accept this disclaimer in full. / We will ask you to agree to this disclaimer before you can access the book.]

(2) Credit

This disclaimer was created using an SEQ Legal template.

(3) No advice

The book contains information about aromatherapy and the use of essential oils.The information is not advice, and should not be treated as such.

[You must not rely on the information in the book as an alternative to qualified medical advice from a health professional. advice from an appropriately qualified professional. If you have any specific questions about any medical matter you should consult an appropriately qualified professional.]

[If you think you may be suffering from any medical condition you should seek immediate medical attention. You should never delay seeking medical advice, disregard medical advice, or discontinue medical treatment because of information in the book.]

(4)   No representations or warranties

To the maximum extent permitted by applicable law and subject to section 6 below, we exclude all representations, warranties, undertakings and guarantees relating to the book.

Without prejudice to the generality of the foregoing paragraph, we do not represent, warrant, undertake or guarantee:

> that the information in the book is correct, accurate, complete or non-misleading;

that the use of the guidance in the book will lead to any particular outcome or result; or

in particular, that by using the guidance in the book you will heal disease or work in any way as a cure for illness.

(5) Limitations and exclusions of liability

The limitations and exclusions of liability set out in this section and elsewhere in this disclaimer: are subject to section 6 below; and govern all liabilities arising under the disclaimer or in relation to the book, including liabilities arising in contract, in tort (including negligence) and for breach of statutory duty.

We will not be liable to you in respect of any losses arising out of any event or events beyond our reasonable control.

We will not be liable to you in respect of any business losses, including without limitation loss of or damage to profits, income, revenue, use, production, anticipated savings, business, contracts, commercial opportunities or goodwill.

We will not be liable to you in respect of any loss or corruption of any data, database or software.

We will not be liable to you in respect of any special, indirect or consequential loss or damage.

(6) Exceptions

Nothing in this disclaimer shall: limit or exclude our liability for death or personal injury resulting from negligence; limit or exclude our liability for fraud or fraudulent misrepresentation; limit any of our liabilities in any way that is not permitted under applicable law; or exclude any of our liabilities that may not be excluded under applicable law.

(7) Severability

If a section of this disclaimer is determined by any court or other competent authority to be unlawful and/or unenforceable, the other sections of this disclaimer continue in effect.

If any unlawful and/or unenforceable section would be lawful or enforceable if part of it were deleted, that part will be deemed to be deleted, and the rest of the section will continue in effect.

(8) Law and jurisdiction

This disclaimer will be governed by and construed in accordance with English law, and any disputes relating to this disclaimer will be subject to the exclusive jurisdiction of the courts of England and Wales.

(9)   Our details

In this disclaimer, "we" means (and "us" and "our" refer to) [*Elizabeth Ashley*] of [*SY8 1LQ*].

Printed in Great Britain
by Amazon.co.uk, Ltd.,
Marston Gate.